DIGITAL RADIOGRAPHY
and PACS

SECOND EDITION

Christi E. Carter, MSRS, RT(R), CIIP
Professor and Director, Radiologic Sciences Program,
Brookhaven College, Farmers Branch, Texas

Beth L. Vealé, Ph.D., RT(R)(QM)
Associate Professor of Radiologic Sciences,
Midwestern State University, Wichita Falls, Texas

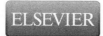

ELSEVIER
MOSBY

3251 Riverport Lane
Maryland Heights, Missouri 63043

DIGITAL RADIOGRAPHY AND PACS   ISBN: 978–0–323–08644–8
Copyright © 2014 by Mosby, an imprint of Elsevier Inc.

Notice

Knowledge and best practice in this field are constantly changing. As new research and experience broaden our knowledge, changes in practice, treatment and drug therapy may become necessary or appropriate. Readers are advised to check the most current information provided (i) on procedures featured or (ii) by the manufacturer of each product to be administered, to verify the recommended dose or formula, the method and duration of administration, and contraindications. It is the responsibility of the practitioner, relying on their own experience and knowledge of the patient, to make diagnoses, to determine dosages and the best treatment for each individual patient, and to take all appropriate safety precautions. To the fullest extent of the law, neither the Publisher nor the Editors/Authors assume any liability for any injury and/or damage to persons or property arising out of or related to any use of the material contained in this book.

                                            The Publisher

Library of Congress Cataloging-in-Publication Data

Carter, Christi E., author.
  Digital radiography and PACS / Christi E. Carter, Beth L. Veale.—Second edition.
    p. ; cm.
  Preceded by Digital radiography and PACS / Christi E. Carter, Beth L. Veal?. Rev. c2010.
  Includes bibliographical references.
  ISBN 978-0-323-08644-8 (pbk. : alk. paper)
  I. Veal?, Beth L., author. II. Title.
  [DNLM: 1. Image Processing, Computer-Assisted—methods. 2. Radiographic Image Enhancement—methods. 3. Radiographic Image Interpretation, Computer-Assisted—instrumentation. 4. Radiographic Image Interpretation, Computer-Assisted—methods. 5. Radiology Information Systems. WN 26.5]
  RC78.7.D35
  616.07′572—dc23
                                           2013021240

Executive Content Strategist: Sonya Seigafuse
Associate Content Development Specialist: Andrea Hunolt
Content Coordinator: Kat Dortch
Publishing Services Manager: Catherine Jackson
Project Manager: Sara Alsup
Design Direction: Theresa McBryan

Printed in the United States of America
Last digit is the print number: 9   8   7   6   5   4

*To our families and colleagues too numerous to name
and to our many students—past, present, and future—
you are the reason this book was written.*

REVIEWERS

Shirley Bartley, M.B.A., RT(R)(N)
Program Coordinator–Radiologic Technology
Hillyard Technical Center
St. Joseph, Missouri

Nan Bradeen, BSRT(R)(M)(QM)
Clinical/Didactic Instructor–Medical
  Radiography
Rapid City Regional Hospital
Rapid City, South Dakota

Carolyn Cianciosa, MSRT
Prior Learning Assessment Instructor
SUNY Empire State College
Niagara Frontier Center
Cheektowaga, New York

Russell H. Crank, M.S., RT(R)
Program Director–Radiologic Technology
Rockingham Memorial Hospital
Harrisonburg, Virginia

Buddy Glidewell, RT(R)(MR)
Clinical Instructor
Southern Union State Community College
Opelika, Alabama

Ann Hagenau, M.S., RT(R)(M)
Assistant Professor–Radiologic Technology and
  Medical Imaging
Clarkson College
Omaha, Nebraska

Clyde Randall Hembree, M.B.A., ARRT(R)
Program Director
University of Tennessee Medical Center, School
  of Radiology
Knoxville, Tennessee

Barbara Jean Kilgore, M.Ed., ARRT(R)
Program Director
Clovis Community College
Clovis, New Mexico

Paul A Kusber, ARRT, RT(R)(CT), CRT
Mills Peninsula School of Diagnostic Imaging
Mills Peninsula Hospital, a Sutter Affiliate
San Mateo, California

Eric Michael Langness, LS-ARRT, Radiography
  A.A.S.
Instructor–Radiologic Technology
Director–Externship/Career Center
Anthem College
St. Louis Park, Minnesota

Deborah R. Leightly, M.Ed., RT(R)(BD)
Clinical Coordinator
Hillsborough Community College
Tampa, Florida

Staci M. Maier, ARRT, RT(R), MHA
Program Director
Holy Cross Hospital, School of Radiology
Silver Spring, Maryland

Marlene May, B.S., RT(R)(QM)
Faculty–Radiologic Technology Program
Pueblo Community College
Pueblo, Colorado

Darryl Mendoza, B.S., RT(R)(MR)
Program Director–MRI
Didactic Instructor–Radiology
Mills-Peninsula Health Services, School of
  Diagnostic Imaging
Burlingame, California

PREFACE

Digital imaging is not new; in fact, it has been in constant development since the 1960s. Despite that, its arrival on the diagnostic imaging scene was a bit of a surprise to most imaging technologists. Computed tomography, magnetic resonance imaging, and ultrasound have used digital imaging techniques for quite some time, but the use of digital imaging in diagnostic radiography is relatively new. Digital imaging has expanded so rapidly in the last few years that it has changed forever the way radiographic examinations are viewed.

Although *Digital Radiography and PACS* is intended for entry-level radiography students, we have discovered that few technologists have nearly enough information to allow them to do the best job they can. This book will benefit anyone with the desire to understand why digital imaging works and how they can provide the best imaging techniques possible for better patient care.

All imaging science professionals can benefit not only from reading this book, but also by suggesting updates and improvements. If the information is as forthcoming as we would like, then perhaps among all of us we can get what we need.

New to This Edition

With the second edition, we have updated all of the technology chapters and have rearranged the text based on suggestions from our peers. Thank you all for your input. We believe this has improved the organization of the textbook while maintaining an easy-to-read collection.

Chapters 1, 2, and 3 are an introduction to digital imaging, image characteristics, and basic processing.

Chapters 4, 5, and 6 describe the various image capture systems available in the current market. We have expanded these chapters and removed all vendor-specific information. Please consult vendor-specific material in the user manuals.

Chapters 7 and 8 cover basic computer and networking information. These chapters will lay a basic foundation for the student with little to no computer or networking knowledge.

Chapters 9 and 10 cover the basic premises of a PACS, including DICOM.

Chapters 11 and 12 discuss suggested quality control and assurance activities for PACS and digital projection radiography systems. Always defer to the specific equipment owner's manual for vendor specific QC/QA activities.

Keep in mind that if our text does not answer your specific questions or problems, always refer back to your manufacturer's documentation for specific equipment and software functions.

Features

This book was written with the reader in mind; hence, we have attempted to present the information as clearly and simply as possible. We have supplemented textual explanations with as many **illustrations, photographs,** and **boxes** as would help illuminate ideas without distracting from concepts. Each chapter includes **Objectives** and **Key Terms** lists to help students focus on what they need to learn and finishes with a **Summary** section and **Chapter Review Questions** to reinforce the readings. To ensure a common language, we have included a **Glossary** and an **Abbreviation Table** to completely define key concepts.

Organization

Chapter 1 starts with a basic overview of the concepts central to the focus of this book, including latent image formation for both conventional and digital image processing, with an introduction to PACs and how digital image processing integrates with digital storage systems.

Chapter 2 provides an overview of the characteristics of a digital image. The concept of a standardized exposure indices is also introduced, along with the definition of several key standard image evaluation criteria.

Chapter 3 delves into image sampling and other basic image processing actions. The chapter also discusses several other basic tools that can be used at a technologist quality control workstation.

Chapter 4 investigates photostimulable storage phosphor systems, with particular attention to how the image is captured, converted, and viewed.

Chapter 5 introduces active matrix flat panel systems. Both indirect and direct conversion systems are explained and a discussion of image artifacts is also presented.

Chapter 6 covers the use of charged couple devices and complementary metal oxide semiconductors in indirect conversion systems. The advantages and disadvantages of these systems are also discussed.

Chapter 7 provides a basic overview of the computer, assuming the reader has no prior knowledge or understanding. The chapter introduces basic computer hardware, monitors, operating systems, and computer uses in radiology.

Chapter 8 introduces the reader to computer networking. This chapter covers network classifications, hardware components, and network topologies. Chapter 8 also introduces DICOM (digital imaging communication in medicine) and HL-7 (health level 7) to provide a better understanding of digital communication within the radiology department.

Chapter 9 begins the study of picture archiving and communication systems (PACSs) with an overview of how a PACS functions and the basic categories of workstations. This chapter covers a simple PACS workflow, showing how the images are moved throughout the department. Also discussed are PACS architectures, common workstation functionality, and several specialty workstation functions.

Chapter 10 introduces the PACS archive. Short-term and long-term archival components are discussed along with their practical uses. Application service providers and disaster recovery area also discussed. Chapter 10 also provides an overview of the following PACS peripherals: film digitizers, film imagers (printers), and CD/DVD burners. Each section provides a basic explanation of operation and common uses.

Chapter 11 discusses the process of ensuring quality in a PACS. The chapter begins with a basic overview of quality terms and theories. This chapter is dedicated to ensuring display quality, whether it be on a monitor or film. Other quality factors, such as speed, data integrity, and training, are also discussed.

Chapter 12 provides a discussion of total quality theory and includes timelines and schedules for daily, weekly, and monthly quality control activities for the technologist, service personnel, and radiation physicist for cassette-less and cassette-based digital radiography. Repeat analysis, problem reporting, and personal responsibility for proper image marking, repeats, and prevention of artifacts are also discussed.

Teaching Aids for the Instructor

Instructor Resources

Helpful instructor resources accompany the text and reside on Evolve. The resources consist of:

- PowerPoint slides to assist in classroom lecture preparation.
- Test Bank, which includes more than 350 questions in ExamView format.
- Electronic Image Collection, which includes all of the images from the text in PowerPoint and JPEG format.
- Lab activities that can be used in the classroom setting to reinforce student learning.
- Answers to the Chapter Review Questions found at the end of each chapter.

Evolve

Evolve is an interactive learning environment designed to work in coordination with *Digital Radiography and PACS, Second Edition.* Instructors may use Evolve to provide Internet-based course components that reinforce and expand on the concepts delivered in class.

Evolve may be used to publish the class syllabus, outlines, and lecture notes; set up "virtual office hours" and email communication; share important dates and information through the online class Calendar; and encourage student participation through Chat Rooms and Discussion Boards. Evolve also allows instructors to post exams and manage their grade books online. For more information, visit http://evolve.elsevier.com/Carter/digital/ or contact an Elsevier sales representative.

We encourage any correspondence regarding the information contained in this textbook. We will strive to provide the most up-to-date information at the time of publication and we hope that you find this information useful in your classroom and throughout your studies. Please feel free to drop either of us an email with your questions, comments, and suggestions.

Christi E. Carter
Brookhaven College
3939 Valley View Lane
Farmers Branch, TX 75244
ccarter@dcccd.edu

Beth L. Vealé
Midwestern State University
3410 Taft Blvd
Bridwell Hall Room 212
Wichita Falls, TX 76308
beth.veale@mwsu.edu

ACKNOWLEDGMENTS

We would like to thank Elsevier for giving us this wonderful opportunity, no matter how painful the process. Christi would also like to thank her family and friends for their encouragement and forgiveness, as all of her extra time was spent in a book or laptop; her friends and colleagues at Brookhaven College for their patience and advice during this process; and her students for inspiring her to finish this task, knowing that it was really all for them. Beth would like to thank Paul and Erin, and most importantly, the students in radiologic science programs that put into practice the principles upon which this book is based. This book is for them. Both of us would like to thank Andrea Hunolt, who jumped in late in the game and kept us in line, and finally, all the folks at Elsevier for their support, encouragement, and guidance.

Christi E. Carter, MSRS, RT(R), CIIP
Beth L. Vealé, Ph.D., RT(R)(QM)

CONTENTS

PART I

Introduction

Introduction to Digital Radiography and PACS

On completion of this chapter, you should be able to:
- Define the term *digital imaging*.
- Explain latent image formation for conventional film/screen radiography.
- Compare and contrast the latent image formation process for storage phosphor, flat panel with thin-film transistor (TFT), and charge-coupled device (CCD) digital imaging systems.
- Explain what a picture archiving and communication system (PACS) is and how it is used.
- Define digital imaging and communications in medicine (DICOM).

KEY TERMS

Digital imaging
Direct capture digital radiography
Flat panel detector (FPD)
Indirect capture digital radiography

Photostimulable phosphor (PSP)
  image capture
Teleradiology

This chapter is intended to present a brief overview of digital imaging and the picture archiving and communication system (PACS); both topics are covered in depth in the chapters that follow. This chapter also presents several basic definitions, compares and contrasts digital and analog imaging, and discusses the historic development of both digital image capture and PACS. It is important to grasp the basic definitions and concepts before moving to the more involved topics because this information will be useful throughout the textbook. Bear in mind that the major focus of this text is on entry-level radiography. Although advanced modalities such as magnetic resonance imaging (MRI), computed tomography (CT), and others may be touched on, this text will not dig deeply into those areas.

CONVENTIONAL FILM/SCREEN RADIOGRAPHY

Before defining and discussing digital imaging, a basic understanding of conventional film/screen imaging must be established. Conventional radiography uses film and intensifying screens in its image formation process. Film is placed on one or between two intensifying screens that emit light when struck by x-rays. The light exposes the film in proportion to the amount and energy of the x-rays incident on the screen. The film is then processed with chemicals, and the manifest image appears on the sheet of film. The film is taken to a radiologist and placed on a lightbox for interpretation. For further review of how conventional radiographic images are created, please consult a radiographic imaging textbook for a more in-depth explanation of this process.

DIGITAL IMAGING

Digital imaging is a broad term. This type of imaging is what allows text, photos, drawings, animations, and video to appear on the World Wide Web. In medicine, one of the first uses of digital imaging was with the introduction of the CT scanner by Godfrey Hounsfield in the 1970s. In the decades since, all of the other imaging modalities have become digital.

The basic definition of **digital imaging** is any imaging acquisition process that produces an electronic image that can be viewed and manipulated on a computer. Most modern medical imaging modalities produce digital images that can be sent through a computer network to various locations.

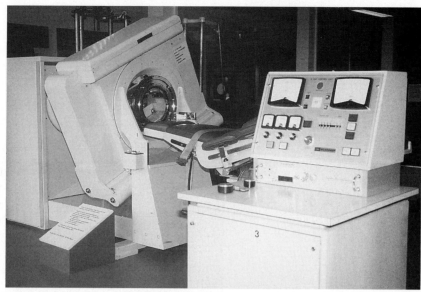

FIGURE 1-1 First-Generation EMI CT Unit: Dedicated Head Scanner. *(Photograph taken at Roentgen Museum, Lennep, Germany.)*

Historical Development of Digital Imaging

CT is second only to the discovery of the x-ray as a major milestone in medical imaging. CT brought about the coupling of the computer and imaging devices. The earliest CT unit built by Hounsfield took several hours to acquire a single slice of information. The machine then took a few days to reconstruct the raw data into a recognizable image. The first commercial CT scanners built were made to image the head only. Figure 1-1 shows one of the early CT scanners built for imaging the head.

MRI was introduced commercially for health care use in the early 1980s. Several companies began pioneering efforts in the mid to late 1970s after the publication of an article by Paul Lauterbur in 1973. Many scientists and researchers were involved in the development of the MRI as we know it today.

Fluoroscopy saw many advances during the 1970s as well thanks to developments in computer technology. Analog-to-digital converters (ADCs) made it possible to capture the images digitally; Plumbicon or Vidicon TV tubes allowed for the display of the dynamic (real-time) image on a television monitor in higher resolution and made it possible to store the frames digitally on a computer. Ultrasound and nuclear medicine were easy converts to the digital world early on because the images created in these modalities were simply frame-grabbed (the current image on the screen is captured and sent as an image file) and converted to a digital image.

DIGITAL RADIOGRAPHY

The concept of moving images digitally was introduced by Albert Jutras in Canada during his experimentation with **teleradiology** (moving images via telephone lines to and from remote locations) in the 1950s. Early PACSs were developed by the

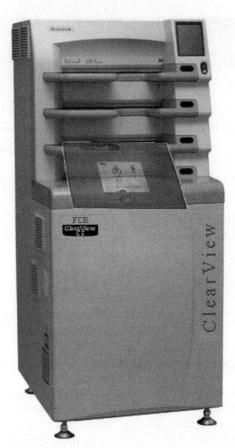

FIGURE 1-2 Fuji PSP Reader, Cassette, and Storage-Phosphor Screen. *(Courtesy FUJIFILM Medical Systems USA, Inc.)*

U.S. military in an effort to move images among Veterans Administration (VA) hospitals and to send battlefield images to established hospitals. These strides were taking place in the early to mid 1980s, and without the government's participation, this technology would not be where it is today. To provide the PACS a digital image, early analog radiographs were scanned into a computer (digitized) so that the images could be sent from computer to computer. The inherently digital modalities were sent via a PACS first, and then as projection radiography technologies advanced, they joined the digital ranks.

Photostimulable Phosphor

Photostimulable phosphor (PSP) image capture (previously known as computed radiography [CR]), is the digital acquisition modality that uses storage phosphor plates to produce projection images. To avoid possible confusion resulting from use of the term *computed*, the technology related to this type of system will be referred to as PSP because the newer systems may or may not be cassette based. PSP imaging can be used in standard radiographic rooms just like film/screen. The only new

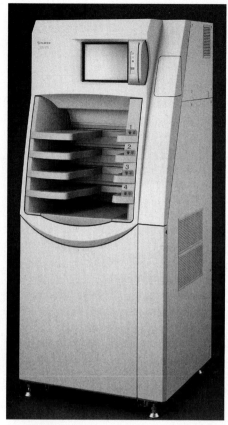 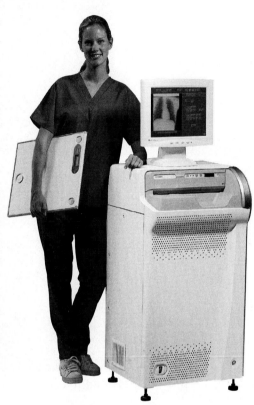

FIGURE 1-3 Examples of Two PSP Readers. **A,** A high-volume reader capable of processing between 110 and 140 imaging plates per hour. **B,** A much smaller system designed for medical offices, surgery, or intensive care units, capable of processing 50 to 60 imaging plates per hour. (**A,** *from Ballinger:* Merrill's atlas, *ed 10, St. Louis, 2003, Mosby;* **B,** *courtesy FUJIFILM Medical Systems USA, Inc.)*

equipment that is required is the PSP and phosphor plates, the PSP readers, the technologist quality control workstation, and a means to view the images, which can be either a printer or a viewing station (Figure 1-2).

The storage phosphor plates are similar to our current intensifying screens. The biggest difference is that the storage phosphors can store a portion of the incident x-ray energy in traps within the material for later readout. More is presented on this topic in Chapter 4.

PSP imaging was first introduced commercially in the United States in 1983 by Fuji Medical Systems of Japan (Figure 1-3). The first system consisted of a phosphor storage plate, a reader, and a laser printer to print the image onto film. PSP imaging did not take off very quickly because many radiologists were reluctant to embrace the new technology. In the early 1990s, PSP imaging began to be installed at a faster rate because of the technological improvements that had occurred in the decade since its introduction. Several major vendors have PSP systems installed in hospitals throughout the United States.

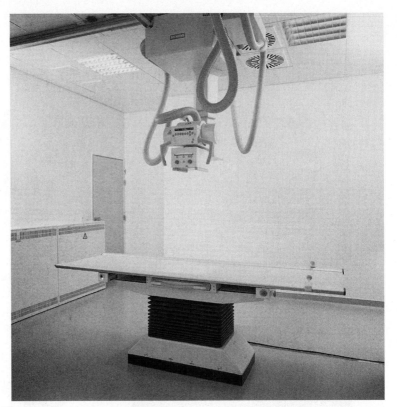

FIGURE 1-4 Axiom Aristos MX FPD Unit. *(Image courtesy of Siemens Healthcare.)*

Flat Panel Detectors

Most **flat panel detector** (FPD) systems use an x-ray absorber material coupled to a thin film transistor or a charge-coupled device (CCD) to form the image. Therefore an existing x-ray room needs to be retrofitted with these devices if a new FPD, TFT, or CCD room is not installed (Figure 1-4).

FPD can be divided into two categories: indirect capture and direct capture. **Indirect capture digital radiography** devices absorb x-rays and convert them into light. The light is then collected by an area-CCD or thin-film transistor (TFT) array and then converted into an electrical signal that is sent to the computer for processing and viewing (Figure 1-5). **Direct capture digital radiography** devices convert the incident x-ray energy directly into an electrical signal, typically using a photoconductor as the x-ray absorber, and send the electrical signal to a TFT and then to an ADC. The ADC signal goes to the computer for processing and viewing (Figure 1-6).

In the early 1970s, several early digital pioneers developed the first clinical application for digital images—digital subtraction angiography (DSA)—at the University of Arizona in Tucson. Drs. M. Paul Capp and Sol Nudelman with Hans Roehrig, Dan Fisher, and Meryll Frost developed the precursor to the current full-field CCD units. As the technology progressed, several companies began developing large field

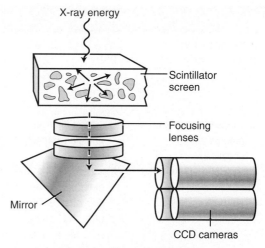

CCD Detector with Scintillator Screen

FIGURE 1-5 The Image Acquisition Process of an Indirect Capture FPD System using CCD Technology.

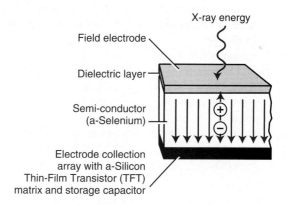

Amorphous Selenium DirectRay Dectector

FIGURE 1-6 The Image Acquisition Process of a Direct Capture FPD System.

detectors, first using the CCD technology developed by the military and shortly thereafter using TFT arrays. CCD and TFT technology developed and continues to develop in parallel. Neither technology has proven to be better than the other.

Again, because of confusion generated by the terms *digital radiography* and *digital imaging* that were the common terms in the past, *FPD* will be used in this text to describe the CCD and TFT technology and *digital imaging* will be used to refer to both PSP and FPD technologies.

TABLE 1-1	Comparison of Conventional, PSP, and FPD		
Factors Considered	**Conventional Radiography**	**PSP**	**FPD**
Imaging room	Traditional x-ray room	Traditional x-ray room	Retrofit traditional x-ray room or install detectors in new room
Ease of use for technologist	Use cassette and film; process with chemicals	Use cassette with phosphor plate; process in PSP reader	No cassette; process at console
Latent image formation	X-rays strike intensifying screen; light is emitted, and film exposed to light	X-rays strike phosphor plate; x-ray energy deposited in the phosphor; energy is released from phosphor when stimulated by light in reader	X-rays strike detector Indirect: phosphor emits light; photodetector (silicon and TFT) detects light and converts to electrical pulse Direct: X-rays detected by photoconductor and converted to electrical signals
Processing	Image processed by chemicals; image appearance based on technical factors and film/screen combination	Image processed by light; image processing takes place in a quality control station based on preset image algorithms	Image detected; image processing takes place at the acquisition console based on preset image algorithms
Exposure response	Nonlinear; narrow exposure latitude	Linear; wide exposure latitude	Linear; wide exposure latitude
Image contrast	kVp and film response curve	kVp and LUTs	kVp and LUTs
Density	mAs	Image processing LUTs	Image processing LUTs
Scatter radiation	Important for patient dose reduction	Important for patient dose reduction and image processing; the phosphor can be more sensitive to low energy photons	Important for patient dose reduction and image processing; the detector can be more sensitive to low energy photons
Noise	Seen with low mAs and fast screens	Seen with inadequate mAs	Seen with inadequate mAs

CR, Computed radiography; *FPD,* Flat panel detector; *kVp,* kilovoltage peak; *LUTs,* look-up tables; *mAs,* milliampere-seconds; *PSP,* Photostimulable phosphor; *TFT,* Thin-film transistor.

Comparison of Film/Screen to PSP and FPD systems

When comparing film/screen imaging with digital projection imaging, several factors should be considered (Table 1-1). For conventional x-ray and PSP systems that use a cassette, a traditional x-ray room with a table and wall Bucky is required. For FPD systems, the detector is located in both the table and wall stand. Because both

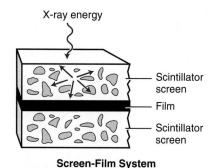

Screen-Film System

FIGURE 1-7 Conventional Radiography Latent Image Formation.

conventional radiography and cassette-based PSP systems use cassettes, technologists often rate them the same in terms of ease and efficiency, but FPD, TFT, and CCD systems have an advantage because the processing is done right at the room's console. The image will appear in 3 to 5 seconds, and the technologist knows right away if the image needs to be repeated. There are cassette-less PSP systems that are faster than the cassette-based PSP system.

Latent image formation is different with conventional radiography (Figure 1-7) and digital projection imaging. In conventional radiographic imaging, a film is placed inside a cassette that contains an intensifying screen. When the x-rays strike the intensifying screen, light is produced. The light photons and x-ray photons interact with the silver halide grains in the film emulsion, and an electron is ejected from the halide. The ejected electron is attracted to the sensitivity speck. The speck now has a negative charge, and silver ions are attracted to equal out the charge. This process happens many times within the emulsion to form the latent image. After chemical processing, the sensitivity specks will be processed into black metallic silver, and the manifest image is formed.

In PSP systems, a photostimulable phosphor plate is placed inside a cassette. Most storage phosphor plates today are made of a barium fluorohalide (where the halide is bromine and/or iodine) with europium as an activator. When x-rays strike the photostimulable phosphor, some light is given off, as in a conventional intensifying screen, but some of the photon energy is deposited within the phosphor particles to create the latent image (Figure 1-8). The phosphor plate is then fed through the PSP reader. To release the latent image, focused laser light (from one or more lasers) is scanned over the plate, causing the electrons to return to their original state and emitting light in the process. This light is picked up by a photomultiplier tube or CCD array and converted into an electrical signal. The electrical signal is then sent through an ADC to produce a digital image that can be sent to the technologist review station.

In FPD the system may be cassette based or cassette-less. The image acquisition device is either built into the table and/or wall stand or enclosed in a portable device. There are two distinct image acquisition methods: indirect capture and direct capture. Indirect capture is very similar to PSP systems in that the x-ray energy stimulates a scintillator, which gives off light that is detected and turned into an

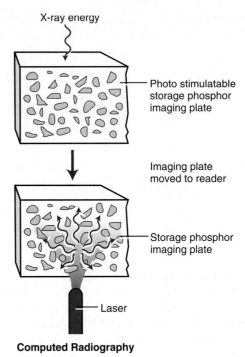

Computed Radiography

FIGURE 1-8 PSP Latent Image Formation.

electrical signal. With direct capture, the x-ray energy is detected by a photoconductor that converts it directly into a digital electrical signal. This process is described in more depth in later chapters.

Image processing in conventional radiography is done with chemicals and the shape of the film's response curve. With digital projection imaging, image processing takes place in a computer. For PSP systems the computer is located near the readers, whether there are several readers distributed throughout the department or there is one centrally located reader. For FPD systems, the computer either is located next to the x-ray console or is integrated within the console, and the image is processed before moving on to the next exposure.

The exposure latitude used in conventional radiography is based on the characteristic response of the film, which is nonlinear. Acquiring images with digital projection imaging, on the other hand, involves using a detector that can respond in a linear manner. The dynamic range is very wide because a single detector can be sensitive to a wide range of exposures. In conventional radiography, radiographic contrast is primarily controlled by kilovoltage peak (kVp). With PSP and FPD systems, kVp still influences subject contrast, but radiographic contrast is primarily controlled by an image processing look-up table (LUT). (A look-up table is a table that maps the image grayscale values into some visible output intensity on a monitor or printed film.) With conventional radiography, optical density on film is primarily controlled by milliampere-seconds (mAs). For digital projection imaging, mAs has more influence on image noise, whereas density is controlled by image processing algorithms (with LUTs). It is important to minimize scattered radiation with all three acquisition systems, but PSP and FPD systems can be more sensitive to scatter than screen/film. The materials used in the many digital projection imaging acquisition devices are more sensitive to low-energy photons.

PICTURE ARCHIVING AND COMMUNICATION SYSTEMS

A PACS is a networked group of computers, servers, and archives that can be used to manage digital images (Figure 1-9). A PACS can accept any image that is in digital imaging and communications in medicine (DICOM) format, for which it is set up to receive, whether it is from cardiology, radiology, or pathology. A PACS serves as the file room, reading room, duplicator, and courier. It can provide image access to multiple users at the same time, on-demand images, electronic annotation of images, and specialty image processing.

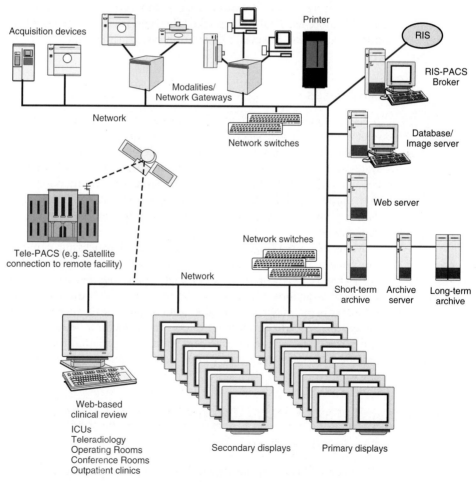

FIGURE 1-9 PACS Network.

A PACS is often custom designed for a facility. The software is generally the same for all PACSs, but the components are arranged differently. Specific factors, such as the volume of patients, the number of areas where images are interpreted, the locations where images are viewed by physicians other than radiologists, and the money available for purchase, are involved in designing a PACS for an institution.

In the early to mid 1980s, different versions of PACS were being developed, primarily by research and academic institutions. They were homegrown and usually involved one or possibly two modalities. These early systems were hard to put together because there was little standardization in image formats. Each vendor had its own proprietary way of archiving images, and there was little need or desire to share archiving methods. Once DICOM (standards that allow imaging modalities and PACS to communicate in the same "language") was established, more vendors began using it to communicate between modalities and PACSs. Pushed by consumer demand, full-scale acceptance of DICOM made it possible for equipment from different manufacturers to communicate with each other. The first full-scale PACS in the United States was installed at the VA Medical Center in Baltimore in 1993. That system covered all modalities except mammography. Soon after installing its PACS, the Baltimore Medical Center asked the vendor to interface to its radiology information system (RIS), hospital information system (HIS), and electronic medical records (EMR).

PACS Uses

A PACS is made up of many different parts, such as the reading stations, physician review stations, web-access, technologist quality control stations, administrative stations, archive systems, and many interfaces to various hospital and radiology systems. Early PACSs were mainly seen in radiology and sometimes in cardiology departments. Now a PACS can receive images from any department in the hospital that sends in a DICOM format for which the PACS has been set up to receive. Archive space (and expense) can now be shared among different hospital departments.

Many PACS reading stations also have image processing capabilities. Radiologists can remain at their workstation and do three-dimensional (3D) reconstructions of a CT (Figure 1-10) or stitch a complete spine together to perform specialized measurement functions for scoliosis. Some PACSs also offer orthopedic workstations for orthopedic surgeons to plan joint replacement surgery before beginning the operation. Specialized software allows the surgeon to load a plain x-ray of the joint and a template for the replacement joint and to match the best replacement to the patient. This software saves a great deal of time in the operating room.

TRANSITIONING FROM FILM/SCREEN TO DIGITAL IMAGING

The Imaging Chain

With both film/screen and digital imaging, the patient is positioned between the x-ray source and the image receptor, image technical and geometric factors are

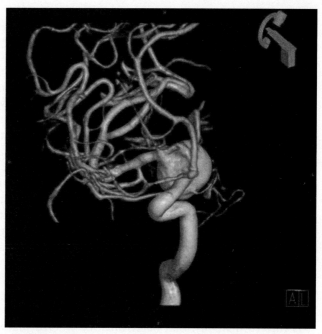

FIGURE 1-10 Three-Dimensional Reconstruction of an Aneurysm. *(Courtesy Siemens Healthcare.)*

selected, and the image captured. However, some differences between the modalities exist, and awareness of these differences can make the transition from film/screen to digital imaging much easier. The specific differences are discussed in more detail in subsequent chapters, but a brief introduction to these follows.

Film versus PSP and FPD

In film/screen imaging, the film is the medium that captures, displays, and archives the image. Phosphor crystals embedded in the film are sensitive to x-ray photons and emit light when the photon strikes an area of sensitivity on the phosphor. After radiation exposure, the film has to be developed through the use of chemicals that develop and fix the image to the film so that it can be viewed with a light source. After review by a radiologist and the generation of a diagnostic report of the findings, the image is stored in a dedicated room and is numbered, lettered, or otherwise physically marked for later retrieval.

Digital image capture occurs by either PSP or FPD systems. The patient is exposed to radiation, and the remnant beam is converted to light then digitized or is sent directly to a computer for conversion to a signal displayed on a computer monitor. The image is given an identification number that ties the image to the patient's medical record. The storage of the resultant image is also through an electronic signal sent to the PACS. Unless printed on film, no physical image is available, and interpretation by the radiologist is electronic as well. Retrieval is accomplished by pulling the image back to a local computer for review.

Patient Demographics

Identification of the patient in film/screen imaging consisted of recording information on a card and then exposing an area of the film after exposure or using lead letters and numbers and placing them on the film for imaging during exposure. Postprocessing labels are applied to indicate such things as patient position, timing, and so on. Proper identification of the patient is even more critical with digital images than with conventional hard copy film/screen images. Retrieval of digital images can be nearly impossible if the images have not been properly and accurately identified. Patient demographics include things such as patient name, health care facility, patient identification number, date of birth, and examination date. This information should be manually entered or linked via barcode label scans before the start of the examination and before the processing phase. Occasionally errors are made, and demographic information must be altered. If the technologist performing the examination is absolutely positive that the image is of the correct patient, then demographic information can be altered at the processing stage. This function should be tracked and changes linked to the technologist altering the information to ensure accuracy and accountability.

Problems arise if the patient name is entered differently from visit to visit or examination to examination. For example, if the patient's name is Jane A. Doe and is entered that way, that name must be entered that way for every other examination. If entered as Jane Doe, the system will save it as a different patient. Merging these files can be difficult, especially if there are several versions of the name. If a patient gives a middle name on one visit but has had multiple examinations under his or her first name, retrieval of previous files will be very difficult and in some cases impossible. The right images must be placed in the correct data files just as hard copy films had to be placed in the correct patient folder.

Technologist Markers

Although digital imaging systems provide a means to add anatomic side identification markers and other demographic information after exposure, every effort must be made to place the anatomic side markers on the image receptor before exposure. Because of the construction of the digital image receptors and related software, images may show on the monitor upside down, backward, or both, making the determination of side (left or right) nearly impossible. Marker errors can result in catastrophic outcomes for patients if used incorrectly.

Technical Choices

The same factors used in film/screen imaging are used in digital imaging. Appropriate selection of mAs, kVp, distance, grids, focal spot size, collimation, and patient protection practices still apply. However, a major difference exists in how the factors affect image capture. Film/screen images are recorded in a logarithmic fashion, whereas digital image capture is linear. What this means to the radiographer is that digital imaging results in a raw image that captures nearly all of the x-ray photons and uses computer software to subtract density values that are outside a predetermined range of diagnostic values for a particular body part. Because of this, higher kVp and lower mAs values can be used without compromising image quality. At the same time, collimation may have to be adjusted; too tight collimation may result in images that indicate underexposure or overexposure when the image is actually acceptable. Because of the increased sensitivity of digital systems to scatter radiation, grid use is more critical to ensure proper image contrast. With recommended higher grid ratios, more accurate grid alignment is required.

Speed

Intensifying screens are used to increase the effect of x-ray photons by conversion of the photons to light in film/screen imaging, resulting in different screen speeds. Slower screens, such as extremity screens, are able to resolve more detail than faster screens; however, faster screens use less radiation, thereby reducing patient dose.

When PSP systems were introduced, a comparison was made to film/screen systems through the term *speed class*, which referred to the PSP's ability to capture the image using certain exposure factors. Many of the first PSP systems had a relative speed, or speed class, of 200. This meant that if a film/screen system had a speed of 400, then the mAs was doubled to compensate. Later, the 15% rule was applied, reducing the exposure to its original intensity. Today, technical factors should change to lower the exposure as much as possible without sacrificing image quality.

Single versus Multiple Exposures

Typically, in film/screen imaging, where multiple images of the same body part are required (such as posteroanterior [PA], oblique, and lateral of the wrist), the images are recorded on the same film. Financially, this made sense because of the high cost of film and because the multiple images per film created an uninterrupted flow for reading and diagnosis. Because there is no physical image material, digital images are usually captured as one per receptor. One reason for doing this is because the image processing software can be compromised if attempting to resolve multiple images. Subsequent image processing allows the single images to be viewed at the same time.

Preparing the Image for Reading

When film/screen imaging systems are used, the processed image is reviewed for errors, and once determined diagnostic, additional labeling occurs. Notes may be attached indicating special circumstances occurring during the examination, patient history relevant to the examination, or explanations for imaging problems. The films are then stored in a particular area for pickup by the radiologist or transported to the radiologist reading area. With digital imaging systems, all relevant information must be attached to the digital file. This can be accomplished by using preset controls such as arrows, position indicators (upright, supine, PA, etc.), or image acquisition markers (cross-table, portable, etc.). Most systems include an option to make notes or annotate the image with text, rules, or other guides.

Getting the Image to the Radiologist

Once the image has been prepared, it must be sent somewhere for the reading radiologist to access. This may be to a dedicated computer in departments without a PACS, where images are stored and archived. Generally, however, images are reviewed on a workstation and then sent to a PACS, where a list is generated for the radiologist to access examinations needing to be read. Images may also be sent to additional workstations for other health care workers to access in areas such as the emergency room, the intensive care or cardiac care units, or surgery.

SUMMARY

- Digital imaging is any imaging acquisition process that produces an electronic image that can be viewed and manipulated on a computer.
- PSP systems are the digital acquisition modality that uses photostimulable phosphor plates to produce digital projection images.
- FPD is divided into two categories: indirect capture and direct capture.
- Indirect capture uses a detector that produces light when struck by x-rays, and then the light is captured and converted to an electrical signal.
- Direct capture uses a detector that captures the x-ray energy and converts it directly to an electrical signal.
- A PACS is a networked group of computers, servers, and archives that can be used to manage digital images.
- DICOM is a standard that allows imaging modalities and PACSs to communicate in the same "language."
- PACSs are made up of many different parts, such as the reading stations, physician review stations, web-access, technologist quality control stations, administrative stations, archive systems, and many interfaces to various hospital and radiology systems.
- Transitioning from film/screen imaging systems to digital imaging systems can be difficult if certain differences are not acknowledged.
- Patient demographics are of equal importance when discussing film/screen or digital image capture. However, it is easier to mark digital images after exposure, which may lead to identification problems. Many different types of preset marking options, as well as measurement and annotations choices, are available with digital imaging systems.
- Technical factor choices have changed in some aspects from film/screen imaging systems to digital imaging systems. Image receptor response has gone from logarithmic to linear, sensitive digital receptors require higher frequency grids, and kVp values are able to be increased and mAs values decreased, reducing patient exposure.

CHAPTER REVIEW QUESTIONS

1. Which radiographic image capture method uses chemical development to produce the manifest image?
   a. Computed tomography
   b. Fluoroscopy

   c. Film/screen radiography

   d. Photostimulable phosphor systems

2. Which company was the first to introduce PSP imaging commercially in the United States?

   a. Carestream (Kodak)

   b. Fuji

   c. Agfa

   d. Konica

3. Which radiographic image capture method uses an x-ray absorber material coupled to a thin film transistor or a charge-coupled device (CCD) to form the digital radiographic image?

   a. PSP

   b. Film/screen

   c. MRI

   d. FPD

4. When x-rays strike a photostimulable phosphor material _____ is released.

   a. Light

   b. Electrons

   c. Heat

   d. Protons

5. The exposure latitude of digital projection radiography responds in a _____ manner.

   a. Nonlinear

   b. Linear

6. The acronym PACS stands for which of the following terms:

   a. Picture arrival computer system

   b. Picture archival computer system

   c. Picture arrival communication system

   d. Picture archiving and communication system

7. In what format must images be in so that they can be sent throughout the image viewing system?

   a. PACS

   b. DICOM

   c. FPD

   d. PSP

8. Patient demographics are unimportant because the RIS will automatically identify all digital images.

   a. True

   b. False

9. Digitally placed anatomic markers can always be used to determine the correct anatomic side of the patient.

   a. True

   b. False

10. Digital systems are less sensitive to scatter radiation than film/screen systems.

   a. True

   b. False

PART II

Basic Principles of Digital Radiography

Digital Imaging Characteristics

KEY TERMS

Air kerma

Analog

Brightness

Contrast resolution

Detective quantum efficiency (DQE)

Deviation index (DI)

Digital

Dynamic range

Field of view (FOV)

Indicated equivalent air kerma (K_{IND})

Latitude

Matrix

Modulation transfer function (MTF)

Noise

Noise power spectrum (NPS)

Pixel

Pixel bit depth

Signal-to-noise ratio (SNR)

Spatial resolution

Standardized radiation exposure (K_{STD})

Target equivalent air kerma value (K_{TGT})

In medical imaging, there are two types of images: analog and digital. Analog images are those types of images that are very familiar to us, such as paintings and printed photographs. What we are seeing in these images are the various levels of brightness and colors; the images are continuous; that is, they are not broken into their individual pieces. **Digital** images are recorded as multiple numeric values and are divided into an array of small elements that can be processed in many different ways.

ANALOG IMAGES VERSUS DIGITAL IMAGES

When we talk about digitizing a signal from a digital radiographic unit, we are talking about assigning a numerical value to each signal point, either an electrical impulse or a light photon. As humans, we experience the world through analog vision. We see our surroundings as infinitely smooth gradients of shapes and colors. **Analog** refers to a device or system that captures or measures a continuously changing signal. In other words, the analog signal wave is recorded or used in its original form. A typical analog device is a watch in which the hands move continuously around the face and is capable of indicating every possible time of day. In contrast, a digital clock is capable of representing only a finite number of times (every tenth of a second, for example).

Traditionally, radiographic images were formed in an analog fashion. A cassette, containing fluorescent screens and film sensitive to the light produced by the screens, is exposed to radiation and then processed in chemical solutions. Today, images can be produced through a digital system that uses detectors to convert the x-ray beam into a digital image.

In an analog system such as film/screen radiography, x-ray energy is converted to light, and the light waves are recorded just as they are. In digital radiography, analog signals are converted into numbers that are recorded. Digital images are formed through multiple samplings of the signal rather than the one single exposure of an analog image.

CHARACTERISTICS OF A DIGITAL IMAGE

A digital image begins as an analog signal. Through computer data processing, the image becomes digitized and is sampled multiple times. The critical characteristics of a digital image are spatial resolution, contrast resolution, noise, and dose efficiency (of the receptor); however, to fully grasp how a digital image is formed, an understanding of its basic components is necessary.

Pixel

A **pixel**, or picture element, is the smallest element in a digital image. If you have ever magnified a digital picture to the point that you see the image as small squares of color, you have seen pixels (Figure 2-1).

Spatially, the digital image is separated into pixels, with discrete (whole numbers only) values. The process of associating the pixels with discrete values defines maximum contrast resolution.

Pixel Size. The size of the pixel is directly related to the amount of spatial resolution or detail in the image. For example, the smaller the pixel is, the greater the detail. Pixel size may change when the size of the matrix or the FOV changes.

Pixel Bit Depth. Each pixel contains pieces or bits of information. The number of bits within a pixel is known as **pixel bit depth**. If a pixel has a bit depth of 8, then

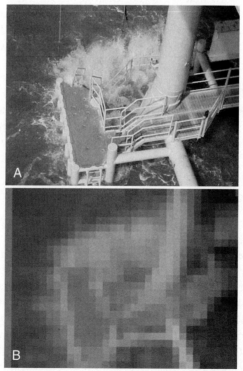

FIGURE 2-1 A, Original image. **B,** Magnified image to display square pixels.

the number of gray tones that pixel can produce is 2 to the power of the bit depth, or 2^8 or 256 shades of gray. Some digital systems have bit depths of 10 to 16, resulting in more shades of gray. Each pixel can have a gray level between 1 (2^0) and 65,536 (2^{16}). The gray level will be a factor in determining the image contrast resolution.

Matrix

A **matrix** is a square arrangement of numbers in columns and rows, and in digital imaging, the numbers correspond to discrete pixel values. Each box within the matrix also corresponds to a specific location in the image and corresponds to a specific area of the patient's tissue. The image is digitized both by position (spatial location) and by intensity (gray level). The typical number of pixels in a matrix ranges from about 512×512 to 1024×1024 and can be as large as 2500×2500. The size of the matrix determines the size of the pixels. For example, if you have a 10×12 and a 14×17 computed radiography (CR) cassette and both have a 512×512 matrix, then the 10×12 cassette will have smaller pixels.

Field of View

The term **field of view**, or FOV, is synonymous with the x-ray field. In other words, it is the amount of body part or patient included in the image. The larger the FOV, the more area is imaged. Changes in the FOV will not affect the size of the matrix; however, changes in the matrix will affect pixel size. This is because as the matrix increases (e.g., from 512×512 to 1024×1024) and the FOV remains the same size, the pixel size must decrease to fit into the matrix (Figure 2-2).

Pixel Size, Matrix Size, and FOV

A relationship may exist between the size of the pixel, the size of the matrix, and the FOV. The matrix size can be changed without affecting the FOV and the FOV can be changed without affecting the matrix size, but a change in either the matrix size and/or the FOV changes the size of the pixels.

Exposure Indicators

The exposure index refers to the amount of exposure received by the image receptor (IR), not by the patient. However, knowing how exposure factors affect the exposure index is key to learning to provide enough exposure to the receptor while limiting exposure to the patient. Because manufacturers differ in the way exposure is numerically represented, it can be difficult to calculate exposure amounts. The clinical world has been calling for exposure indicator standardization for several years. In 2008 the International Electrotechnical Commission (IEC) published a report titled "Medical Electrical Equipment—Exposure Index of Digital X-Ray Imaging Systems—Part 1: Definitions and Requirements for General Radiography," and in 2009 the American Association of Physicists in Medicine (AAPM) released its "An Exposure Indicator for Digital Radiography" report. The AAPM report expressed

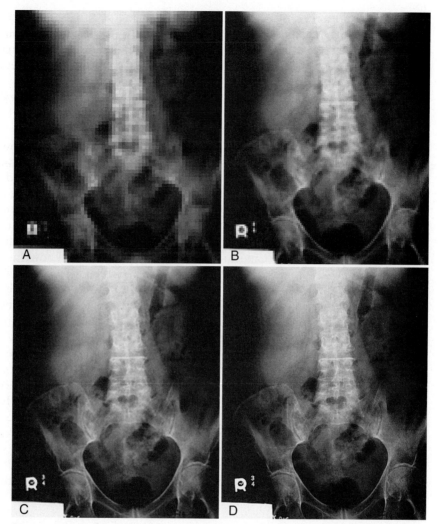

FIGURE 2-2 For a given field of view, the larger the matrix size, the greater the number of smaller individual pixels. Increasing the number of smaller pixels will improve the quality of the image. **A,** Matrix size is 64 × 64. **B,** Matrix size is 215 × 215. **C,** Matrix size is 1024 × 1024. **D,** Matrix size is 2048 × 2048. *(From Fauber TL:* Radiographic imaging and exposure, *ed 3, St. Louis, 2009, Mosby.)*

the clinical need to have this standardization, saying that standardization will give the technologist more confidence in adjusting technical factors while following the ALARA (as low as reasonably achievable) principle. The following paragraphs explain some of the most important terms that came from this research. Further information may be gained about this standardization effort by downloading the AAPM report (No. 116) from the AAPM website. For information on proprietary exposure indices, either contact the vendor directly or consult the equipment manual for specific information.

Standard Units of Measure

Standardized Radiation Exposure (K*_{STD}*). Before the standard radiation exposure is explained, let's first revisit a few radiation units. **Air kerma** (*k*inetic *e*nergy *r*eleased per unit *ma*ss [of air]) is the measurement of radiation energy (joules or J) absorbed in a unit of air (kg). Therefore the quantity kerma is expressed as J/kg or gray (Gy). The gray will be used most often in equipment to express this measurement. When an exposure is made of an IR, the air kerma can be easily read during the processing of the exposure.

The **standardized radiation exposure** (K_{STD}) is a standard exposure typical of that imaging receptor system. The exposure is made with additional filtration that hardens the beam to simulate patient tissue. These standard conditions for the exposure are used to ensure that the equipment is functioning appropriately.

Indicated Equivalent Air Kerma (K*_{IND}*). The **indicated equivalent air kerma** (K_{IND}) is the measurement of the radiation that was incident on the IR for that particular exposure. This measurement is derived from reading the pixel values produced by the exposure on an IR. These values are known as for-processing pixel values (Q), and the median is found after certain data correction has taken place and the median value is then compared to the K_{STD} exposure to derive the K_{IND}. This may seem complicated, but the K_{IND} can be simply stated as the amount of exposure on the IR. This value will help determine whether the IR has been overexposed or underexposed for that particular body part.

Target Equivalent Air Kerma Value (K*_{TGT}*). The **target equivalent air kerma value** (K_{TGT}) is a set of values, established by either the system manufacturer or the system user, that represents an optimal exposure for each specific body part and view. For example, there will be established perfect exposures for a posteroanterior (PA) chest, lateral chest, portable chest, pediatric chest, and so on. Each body part and view will have its own unique optimal exposure. These exposures are listed in a table within the system by body part (b) and view (v), K_{TGT} (b,v).

Deviation Index. The **deviation index** (DI) is simply the difference between the actual exposure (K_{IND}) and the target exposure (K_{TGT}), except that it is expressed in a logarithmic fashion:

$$DI = 10 * \log 10 \left[\frac{K_{IND}}{K_{TGT(b,v)}} \right].$$

The DI is intended to help the technologist determine whether the image has been underexposed or overexposed. Just as with the other exposure indices, the DI is not an end all, be all indicator. Technologists must evaluate the image and, if in doubt about the image's quality, consult with a radiologist. The radiologist has a higher-quality display than what is normally used for technologist workstations; an image that looks fine at the technologist's workstation might show a great deal of noise and unwanted image interference at the radiologist's workstation.

The DI can be used to adjust technical factors if the image must be repeated. A perfect image according to the DI has a DI value of 0.0. If the DI is negative, the image has been underexposed. If the DI is positive, the image has been overexposed. To raise the DI +1, increase technique by 20%. To decrease DI −1, decrease technique by 25%. This ±1 changes the K_{IND} by +25% or −20%. This can also be expressed by saying that +1 is approximately 125% of the intended exposure; −1 is 80% of the intended exposure.

Do not rely on the DI as the sole determining factor of image quality. There are several variances that could cause the reading of the pixel values (Q) to be off, including the following:

- A prostheses within the image
- Gonadal shielding within the image
- Failure of the system to recognize the collimated border
- An unexpected body part in the image

Any of these factors will cause the DI to fluctuate, and the technologist should consult with the radiologist regarding these image variances. The technologist should continue to use image noise as the true determining factor of image acceptance, and these standard values should be used only as a guide.

IMAGE QUALITY CHARACTERISTICS

Brightness

The **brightness** of a digital image refers to its appearance on the display monitor of the computer. The amount of light transmitted by the monitor as well as light reflected off the monitor can affect image appearance. According to the AAPM (Medical Physics Monograph No. 30), a monochromatic monitor uses a single electron beam and will have some overlap from line to line, and be susceptible to drift. In addition, if a monitor is monochromatic, reflection of the light in the room can be a problem. The phosphors produce white light that, when a clear glass monitor is used, the phosphor light escapes the monitor at a high rate. Ambient light is both reflected off the glass and penetrates the glass and reflects back, producing glare. To reduce glare, cathode ray tube (CRT) monitors are tinted so that the emitted light is decreased, and the faceplate glass is flat so that internal reflections are minimized. Controls are available to adjust the brightness of the computer monitor to minimize these issues.

When viewing images in any monitor, the technologist can adjust the brightness of the image using a technique called window level. Changing the window level makes the image brighter or darker. Manipulation of image brightness is discussed further in Chapter 3.

Contrast Resolution

Contrast resolution refers to the ability of the digital system to display subtle changes in the shade of gray. Higher-contrast resolution means that the differences between adjacent densities are enhanced; that is, more shades of gray may be demonstrated, resulting in the ability to differentiate between small differences in densities. Contrast resolution in digital imaging is directly related to the bit depth of the pixels in the image. With digital imaging, higher kilovoltage peak (kVp) values and lower milliampere-seconds (mAs) values can be used, lowering patient dose without affecting contrast nearly as much as was seen in film/screen radiography.

What contrast resolution in digital imaging does depend on is the amount of scatter. Digital systems are much more sensitive in recording scatter; therefore control of scatter is critical. Use of tight collimation and the correct grid will allow higher kVp values to be used without compromising contrast resolution. However, if contrast is too low it can be difficult, if not impossible, to separate the image signal from noise and background. Sufficient kVp for appropriate penetration of the tissues is still required so that enough gray tones exist to provide that signal separation. Screen resolution can be controlled by a technique called window width, in which the displayed tones are varied toward a longer or shorter scale. This is discussed further in Chapter 3.

Spatial Resolution

The ability of the imaging system to demonstrate small details of an object is known as **spatial resolution**. Just as the crystal size and thickness of the phosphor layer determines resolution in film/screen radiography, phosphor layer thickness and pixel size determines resolution in photostimulable phosphor (PSP) systems. The thinner the phosphor layer is, the higher the resolution. In film/screen radiography, resolution at its best is limited to approximately 10 line pairs per millimeter (lp/mm). In digital receptors, resolution is approximately 2.55 lp/mm up to 10 lp/mm in PSP systems, resulting in less detail. However, because of the **dynamic range,** or the ability to respond to varying levels of exposure, more tissue densities on the digital image are seen, giving the appearance of more detail. For example, an anteroposterior (AP) knee film/screen radiograph typically does not show soft tissue structures on the lateral aspects of the distal femur or proximal tibia or fibula. An AP knee digital image shows not only the soft tissue but also the edge of the skin (Figure 2-3). This is because of the wider dynamic recording range and does not mean there is additional detail. Spatial resolution comes down to this: the smaller the pixels, the higher the spatial resolution.

MODULATION TRANSFER FUNCTION

To quantify gain or loss of resolution, a mathematical theorem was developed that stated that spatial resolution can be broken down into individual components and that the quality of each component affects the total amount of resolution. The ability of a system to record available spatial frequencies is known as **modulation transfer function (MTF).** The sum of the components in a recording system cannot be greater than the system as a whole. What that means is that when any component's function is compromised because of some type of interference, the overall quality of the system is affected. MTF is a way to quantify the contribution of each system component to the overall efficiency of the entire system. MTF is a ratio of the image to the object; thus a perfect system would have an MTF of 1 or 100%. In digital detectors where x-ray photon energy excites a phosphor/scintillation layer and that phosphor produces light, there will always be a spreading out of the light that will reduce system efficiency; therefore the more light spread there is, the less the image looks like the object and the lower the MTF will be (Figure 2-4).

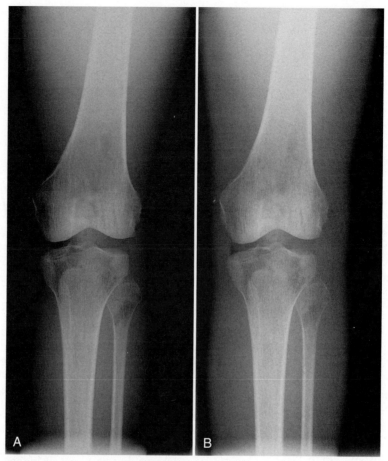

FIGURE 2-3 A, Film/screen AP knee radiograph. **B,** Digital AP knee image. Note the differences in the amount of soft tissue shown in detail.

Noise

Both in film/screen and digital imaging, anything that interferes with the formation of the image is considered **noise**. If superimposition of body parts occurs, that is known as anatomic noise. Noise that occurs during the acquisition of the image is known as radiographic noise and comprises equipment noise and quantum noise.

Equipment noise comes from noise in the detector elements and non-uniform detector responses. This cannot be controlled by the radiographer and is highly dependent on manufacturer, technology, and detector quality.

To place a relative value on noise, the **noise power spectrum (NPS)** is used. The NPS describes the spatial frequency content of the noise as well as spatial characteristics. The higher the NPS, the higher the noise is for a specific detector. Measuring NPS requires uniform exposures at specified beam qualities and exposures, followed by sophisticated mathematical measurements, the discussion of which is beyond the scope of this book.

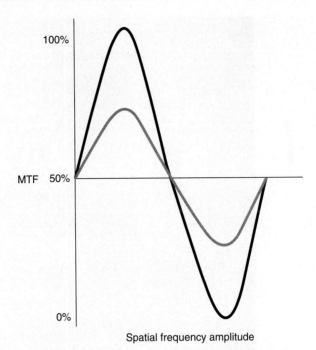

100%

MTF   50%

0%

Spatial frequency amplitude

FIGURE 2-4 **MTF Comparison.** The black line shows high spatial frequency, which results in an MTF of 100%. The gray line shows a substantially lower spatial frequency, indicating system inefficiency. The closer the amplitude of the spatial frequency is to becoming a flat line, the lower the MTF.

When determining the appropriate exposure techniques to use for a particular body part, it must be decided by the radiologist and technologist how much noise can be tolerated in the image. This is known as **signal-to-noise ratio (SNR)**. As the SNR increases, the noise decreases, but at a cost of higher exposure to the patient. Different detectors will require more or less exposure to the IR to achieve the same SNR. This can be difficult if there are multiple types of equipment from multiple vendors represented in one department. This is the reason for the push for a standardized exposure indicator mentioned earlier in the chapter.

Exposure Latitude

Latitude refers to the range of exposure diagnostic image values the image detector is able to produce. It is those values that are just above background noise and higher and that refer to how much signal amplification is needed. Latitude is dependent on the image detector; the higher the dynamic range of the detector, the more values can be detected. In addition to the range of exposures and the way the detector responds within that range, images must have sufficient contrast resolution for the signal to be detected. The signal from the anatomic part must be appropriate and provide enough gray level so that its signal can be separated from background and noise. For example, when a homogenous object is x-rayed, there will be no contrast resolution, but when a heterogeneous object is x-rayed, there will be a great difference in adjacent tissues (Figure 2-5).

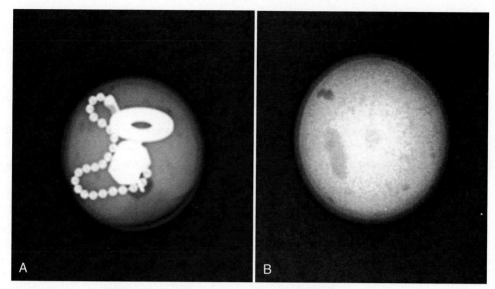

FIGURE 2-5 A, Homogenous object. **B,** Heterogeneous object.

Detective Quantum Efficiency

How efficiently a system converts the x-ray input signal into a useful output image is known as **detective quantum efficiency (DQE)**. DQE is a measurement of the percentage of x-rays that is absorbed when they hit the detector. The linear, wide-latitude input/output characteristic of PSP systems relative to screen/film systems leads to a wider DQE latitude for PSP systems, which implies that a PSP has the ability to convert incoming x-rays into "useful" output over a much wider range of exposures than can be accommodated with screen/film systems. Systems with higher quantum efficiency can produce higher-quality images at lower doses.

Amorphous selenium, amorphous silicon thin-film transistor (TFT), charge-coupled device (CCD), and complementary metal oxide semiconductor detector technology have increased DQE over PSP. Amorphous selenium detectors have the highest DQE, because they do not have the light conversion step and consequently no light spread. There is no light to blur the recorded signal output, a lower dose is required than for the others, and higher-quality images are produced. Newer complementary metal oxide semiconductor (CMOS) capture systems may be equal to direct image acquisition because of the crystal light tubes, which also prevent light spread.

The DQE of detectors changes with kVp, but generally the DQE of selenium systems is higher than that for PSP, CCD, and CMOS systems. CCD in particular has problems with low light capture.

The area of a TFT array is limited because of the structure of the matrix. This also affects the size and number of pixels available. Known as the fill factor, the larger the area of the TFT photodiodes, the more radiation can be detected and the greater amount of signal generated. Consequently, the greater the area of the TFT array, the higher the DQE.

SUMMARY

- Two types of images exist in radiography: analog and digital. Analog images are those that are made up of continuous, varied levels of brightness and colors.
- Analog capture of an image involves the measurement of a continuously changing signal. Digital image capture represents a finite number of bits of information.
- For analog systems, x-ray energy is converted to light and recorded on film. In digital, multiple samples of the signal are taken.
- Digital images begin as analog signals that are recorded and turned into electrical signals, then digitized.
- Digital images consist of pixels, which can be different sizes and shades of gray. The smaller the pixel, the greater number of pixels can be used for an image, and the greater the depth, the more shades of gray can be recorded.
- Pixels are arranged in columns and rows called a matrix. The larger the matrix, the smaller the pixels.
- *Field of view* refers to the amount of patient tissue included in the image. The larger the FOV, the more body area imaged. Matrix size can be changed without affecting the FOV; however, changes in the matrix size or the FOV affect pixel size.
- *Brightness* is a term used to describe the image appearance on the computer monitor. Reflected and transmitted light from the monitor can affect image appearance, especially if the monitor is monochromatic. To decrease the problems of glare and reflection, monitor faceplate glass is tinted.
- *Contrast resolution* refers to the digital system's ability to demonstrate subtle differences in gray shades, especially those in adjacent structures. It is a direct result of pixel bit depth, allowing higher kVp and lower mAs values. Because digital recording media are so sensitive, more values, including scattered photons, are recorded so that scatter control becomes critical.
- Spatial resolution is the ability to distinguish small structures from background and noise. Film/screen imaging is able to produce resolution up to 10 lp/mm, whereas digital images are able to resolve only about 2.5 to 5 lp/mm and PSP systems as much as 10 lp/mm. Because of their wider dynamic ranges, digital images appear to have greater spatial resolution, but in reality, they do not.
- *Modulation transfer function* refers to the ability of combined components of a system to accurately reproduce the structural details of an object within the image. Resolution will be limited to the component that produces the least resolution.
- Anatomy and equipment can cause noise on digital images. Anatomic noise can be controlled by the radiographer while equipment noise usually cannot. However, failure to properly maintain equipment such as digital receptors that become dirty or have not been erased is within the control of the radiographer.
- Latitude, or the range of exposures a digital detector can respond to, depends on the detector and the available contrast resolution.
- Detective quantum efficiency measures the efficiency of a system to convert the x-ray input signal into a useful output image.

CHAPTER REVIEW QUESTIONS

1. An image formed by recording a continuous changing signal is known as:
   a. Photographic
   b. Digital
   c. Analog
   d. Electric

2. The arrangement of pixels in rows and columns is known as:
   a. Pixelation
   b. Matriculation
   c. Matrix
   d. Spatial

3. The amount of tissue included in the image is referred to as:
   a. Collimation
   b. Field of view
   c. Inclusion
   d. Digital view

4. The measurement of the radiation that was incident on the image receptor for a particular exposure is known as:
   a. K_{STD}
   b. K_{IND}
   c. K_{TGT}
   d. DI

5. The difference between the actual exposure and the target exposure is known as the:
   a. K_{STD}
   b. K_{IND}
   c. K_{TGT}
   d. DI

6. Contrast resolution is a digital system's ability to:
   a. Record noise interference
   b. Separate structures from noise
   c. Show small differences in gray levels
   d. Allow lower kVp and higher mAs values

7. Dynamic range is the ability of a digital imaging system to respond to varying levels of exposure.
   a. True
   b. False

8. Spatial resolution in digital imaging is dependent on pixel size.
   a. True
   b. False

9. The best component in a digital system will determine the resolution in a digital image.
   a. True
   b. False

10. Which of the following measures the efficiency of a system to convert the x-ray input signal into a useful output image?
a. MTF
b. DQE
c. Exposure latitude
d. Spatial resolution

Digital Radiographic Image Processing and Manipulation

OBJECTIVES

On completion of this chapter, you should be able to:
- Describe the formation of an image histogram.
- Discuss automatic rescaling.
- Compare image latitude in digital imaging with film/screen radiography.
- List the functions of contrast enhancement parameters.
- State the Nyquist theorem.
- Describe the effects of improper algorithm application.
- Discuss the purpose and function of image manipulation factors.
- Describe the major factors in image management.

OUTLINE

KEY TERMS

Aliasing

Archive query

Automatic rescaling

Contrast manipulation

Critical frequency

Edge enhancement

High-pass filtering

Histogram

Image annotation

Image orientation

Image sampling

Image stitching

Look-up table (LUT)

Low-pass filtering

Manual send

Nyquist theorem

Patient demographics

Shuttering

Smoothing

Spatial frequency resolution

Window level

Window width

Once x-ray photons have been converted into electrical signals, these signals are available for processing and manipulation. This is true for both photostimulable phosphor (PSP) systems and flat-panel detector (FPD) systems, although a reader is used only for PSP systems. Processing parameters and image manipulation controls are also similar for both systems.

Preprocessing takes place in the computer where the algorithms determine the image histogram. Postprocessing is done by the technologist through various user functions. Digital preprocessing methods are vendor specific, so only general information on this topic can be covered here.

PSP READER FUNCTIONS

The PSP imaging plate records a wide range of x-ray exposures. If the entire range of exposure were digitized, values at the extremely high and low ends of the exposure range would also be digitized, resulting in low-density resolution. To avoid this, exposure data recognition processes only the optimal density exposure range. The data recognition program searches for anatomy recorded on the imaging plate by finding the collimation edges and then eliminates scatter outside the collimation. Failure of the system to find the collimation edges can result in incorrect data collection, and images may be too bright or too dark. It is equally important to center the anatomy to the center of the imaging plate. This also ensures that the appropriate recorded densities will be located. Failure to center the imaging plate may also result in an image that is too bright or too dark. The data within the collimated area produce a graphic representation of the optimal densities called a **histogram** (Figure 3-1). The value of each tone is represented (horizontal axis), as is the number of pixels in each tone (vertical axis). Values at the left represent black areas. As tones vary toward the right, they get brighter, with the middle area representing medium tones. The extreme right area represents white. A dark image will show the majority of its data points on the left, and a light image will show the majority of its data points on the right.

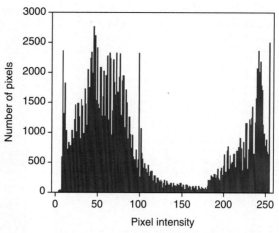

FIGURE 3-1 Simple Histogram Illustration. A graphical representation of the number of pixels with a particular intensity.

Because the information within the collimated area is the signal that will be used for image data, this information is the source of the vendor-specific exposure data indicator.

IMAGE SAMPLING

With **image sampling**, the plate is scanned and the image's location is determined. The size of the signal is then determined, and a value is placed on each pixel. A histogram is generated from the image data, which allows the system to find the useful signal by locating the minimum (S1) and maximum (S2) signal within the anatomic regions of interest on the image and then plots the intensities of the signal on a histogram. The histogram identifies all intensities on the imaging plate in the form of a graph on which the *x*-axis is the amount of exposure read, and the *y*-axis is the number of pixels for each exposure. This graphic representation appears as a pattern of peaks and valleys that varies for each body part. Low energy (low kilovoltage peak [kVp]) gives a wider histogram; high energy (high kVp) gives a narrower histogram. The histogram shows the distribution of pixel values for any given exposure. For example, if pixels have a value of 1, 2, 3, and 4 for a specific exposure, then the histogram shows the frequency (how often they occurred) of each of those values, as well as the actual number of values (how many were recorded).

Analysis of the histogram is very complex. However, it is important to know that the shape of the histogram is anatomy specific, which is to say that it stays fairly constant for each part exposed. For example, the shape of a histogram generated from a chest x-ray on an adult patient will look very different than a knee histogram generated from a pediatric knee examination. This is why it is important to choose the correct anatomic region on the menu before processing the image plate. The raw data used to form the histogram are compared with a "normal" histogram of

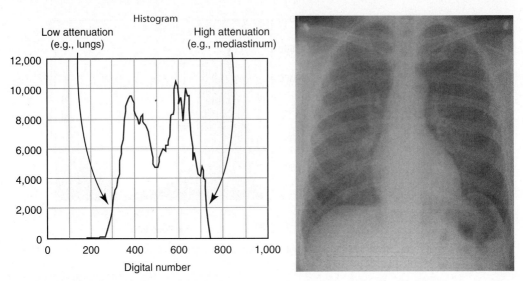

FIGURE 3-2 The histogram shows the pixel values found within this chest x-ray. *(Courtesy American Association of Physicists in Medicine.)*

the same body part by the computer, and the image correction takes place at this time (Figure 3-2).

DIGITAL RADIOGRAPHY IMAGE SAMPLING

The Nyquist Theorem

In 1928 Harry Nyquist, who was a researcher for AT&T, published the paper "Certain Topics in Telegraph Transmission Theory." He described a way to convert analog signals into digital signals that would more accurately transmit over telephone lines. He found that since an analog signal was limited to specific high frequencies, it could be captured and transmitted digitally and recreated in analog form on the receiver. He said that the sampling rate would need to be at least twice the highest frequency to be reproduced. In 1948 Claude Shannon presented a mathematical proof of Nyquist's theory, allowing it to be called the Nyquist theorem. Since that time, a number of scientists have added to and revised the theory. In fact, it could be called the Nyquist–Shannon–Kotelnikov, Whittaker–Shannon–Kotelnikov, Whittaker–Nyquist–Kotelnikov–Shannon (WNKS), etc., sampling theorem, as well as the Cardinal Theorem of Interpolation Theory. It is often referred to simply as the sampling theorem.

The **Nyquist theorem** states that when sampling a signal (such as the conversion from an analog image to a digital image), the sampling frequency must be greater than twice the frequency of the input signal so that the reconstruction of the original image will be as close to the original signal as possible. In digital imaging, at least twice the number of pixels needed to form the image must be sampled. If too few pixels are sampled, the result will be a lack of resolution. At the same time, there is a point at which oversampling does not result in additional useful information. Once the human eye can no longer perceive an improvement in resolution, there is no need for additional sampling.

The number of conversions that occur in PSP imaging—electrons to light, light to digital information, digital to analog signal—results in loss of detail. Light photons do not travel in one direction, so some light will be lost during the light-to-digital conversion because light photons spread out. Because there is a small distance between the phosphor plate surface and the photosensitive diode of the photomultiplier, some light will spread out there as well, resulting in loss of information. In addition, even though the imaging plate is able to store electrons for an extended period of time, the longer the electrons are stored, the more energy they lose. When the laser stimulates these electrons, some of the lower energy electrons will escape the active layer, but if enough energy was lost, some lower energy electrons will not be stimulated enough to escape and information will be lost. All manufacturers suggest that imaging plates be read as soon as possible to avoid this loss.

Although FPD systems lose fewer signals to light spread than PSP systems, the Nyquist theorem is still applied to ensure that sufficient signal is sampled. Because the sample is preprocessed by the computer immediately, signal loss is minimized but still occurs.

Aliasing

When the spatial frequency is greater than the Nyquist frequency and the sampling occurs less than twice per cycle, information is lost and a fluctuating signal is produced. When the signal is reproduced, frequencies above the Nyquist frequency cause **aliasing**. This is also known as foldover or biasing, and causes mirroring of the signal at $\frac{1}{4}$ the frequency. A wraparound image is produced, which appears as two superimposed images that are slightly out of alignment, resulting in a moiré effect. This can be problematic because the same effect can occur with grid errors. It is important for technologists to look at both.

Additionally, when a sampled frequency is exactly at the Nyquist frequency, often a zero amplitude signal will result. This is called the **critical frequency** and results from frequency phase shifts, causing aliasing of the signal.

Automatic Rescaling

When exposure is greater or less than what is needed to produce an image, automatic rescaling occurs in an effort to display the pixels for the area of interest. **Automatic rescaling** means that images are produced with uniform density and contrast, regardless of the amount of exposure. Problems occur with rescaling when too little exposure is used, resulting in quantum mottle, or when too much exposure is used, resulting in loss of contrast and loss of distinct edges because of increased scatter production. Rescaling is no substitute for appropriate technical factors. There is a danger in relying on the system to "fix" an image through rescaling and in the process using higher milliamperage seconds (mAs) values than necessary to avoid quantum mottle. The term *dose creep* is widely used to explain

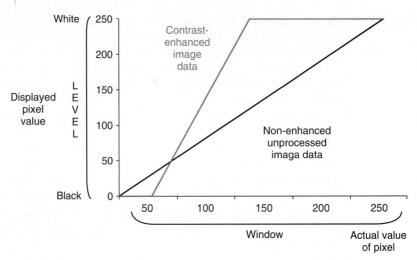

FIGURE 3-3 Look-Up Table. Gray-level transformation required for contrast enhancement of images with 256 shades of gray for an 8-bit matrix. The nonenhanced image data are transformed so that data with pixel values less than 50 are displayed as black, and all data with pixel values greater than 150 are displayed as white. All data with pixel values between 50 and 150 are displayed using an intermediate shade of gray.

this phenomenon. It refers to the use of automatic rescaling without regard to appropriate exposure amount. What may be appropriate for one patient may be too much exposure for another; however, the same factors are used. Therefore the dose "creeps" up over time.

Look-Up Table

A **look-up table** (LUT) is a histogram of the luminance values derived during image acquisition. The LUT is used as a reference to evaluate the raw information and correct the luminance values. This is a mapping function in which all pixels (each with its own specific gray value) are changed to a new gray value. The resultant image will have the appropriate appearance in brightness (density) and contrast. There is an LUT for every anatomic part. The LUT can be graphed by plotting the original values ranging from 0 to 255 on the horizontal axis and the new values (also ranging from 0 to 255) on the vertical axis. Contrast can be increased or decreased by changing the slope of this graph. The brightness (density) can be increased or decreased by moving the line up or down the y-axis (Figure 3-3).

QUALITY CONTROL WORKSTATION FUNCTIONS

Image Processing Parameters

As previously discussed, digital systems have a greater dynamic range than film/screen imaging. The initial digital image appears linear when graphed because all shades of gray are visible, giving the image a very wide latitude. If all of the shades were left in the image, the contrast would be so low as to make adjacent densities difficult to differentiate. To avoid this, digital systems use various contrast enhancement parameters. Although the parameter names differ by vendor (Agfa [Mortsel, Belgium] uses MUSICA; Fuji [Tokyo, Japan] uses Gradation; and Kodak uses Tonescaling), the purpose and effects are basically the same.

Contrast Manipulation

Contrast manipulation involves converting the digital input data to an image with appropriate brightness and contrast using contrast enhancement parameters. Image contrast is controlled by using a parameter that changes the steepness of the exposure gradient. By using a different parameter, the brightness can be varied at the toe and shoulder of the curve to remove the extremely low values and the extremely high values. Another parameter allows brightness to remain unchanged, whereas contrast is varied. These parameters should be used only to enhance the image. No amount of adjustment can take the place of proper technical factor selection (Figure 3-4).

Spatial Frequency Resolution

Detail or sharpness is referred to as **spatial frequency resolution**. In film/screen radiography, sharpness is controlled by various factors such as focal spot size, screen and/or film speed, and object-image distance (OID). Focal spot and the OID affect image sharpness in both film/screen and digital imaging. The digitized image, however, can be further controlled for sharpness by adjusting processing parameters. The technologist can choose the structure to be enhanced, control the degree of enhancement for each density to reduce image graininess, and adjust how much edge enhancement is applied. Great care must be taken when making adjustments to processing parameters because if the improper algorithms are applied, image formation can be degraded.

Many health care facilities do not want the technologist to manipulate the image much before it goes to the picture archiving and communication system (PACS) because their changes reduce the amount of manipulation that the radiologist can do. Once the image is stored in the PACS, all postprocessing activities result in a loss of information from the original image.

Spatial Frequency Filtering

Edge Enhancement. After the signal is obtained for each pixel, the signals are averaged to shorten processing time and storage. The more pixels involved in the averaging, the smoother the image appears. The signal strength of one pixel is averaged with the strength of adjacent pixels, or neighborhood pixels. **Edge enhancement** occurs when fewer pixels in the neighborhood are included in the signal average. The smaller the neighborhood, the greater the enhancement is. When the frequencies of areas of interest are known, those frequencies can be amplified and other frequencies suppressed. This is also known as **high-pass filtering** and increases

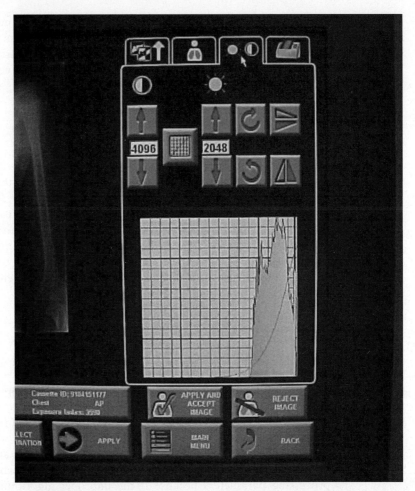

FIGURE 3-4 Workstation screen showing contrast manipulation choices.

contrast and edge enhancement. Suppressing frequencies, also known as *masking*, can result in the loss of small details. High-pass filtering is useful for enhancing large structures such as organs and soft tissues, but it can be noisy (Figure 3-5).

Smoothing. Another type of spatial frequency filtering is **smoothing**. Also known as **low-pass filtering**, smoothing occurs by averaging each pixel's frequency with surrounding pixel values to remove high-frequency noise. The result is a reduction of noise and contrast. Low-pass filtering is useful for viewing small structures such as fine bone tissues.

BASIC FUNCTIONS OF THE PROCESSING SYSTEM

Image Manipulation

Window and Level. The most common image processing parameters are those for brightness and contrast. **Window level** controls how bright or dark the screen

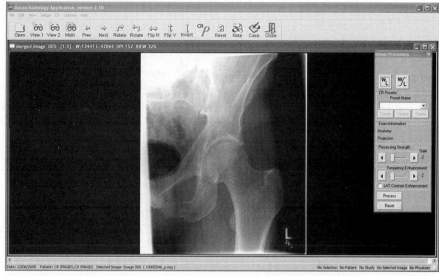

A

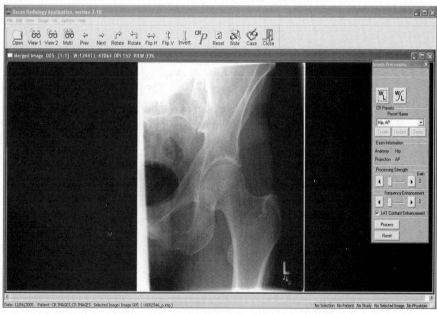

B

FIGURE 3-5 Edge Enhancement. A, AP hip image without edge enhancement. **B,** The same AP hip image with edge enhancement.

image is, and **window width** controls the ratio of black and white, or contrast. The higher the level is, the darker the image will be, and the wider the window width, the lower the contrast. The user can quickly manipulate both by using the mouse. One direction (vertical or horizontal) controls brightness, and the other direction controls contrast. Remember, windowing and leveling are manipulations of the screen image and are not adding or subtracting radiation exposure to the patient. Minimal manipulation will be required on an image with appropriate exposure factors. To further control brightness and contrast, contrast enhancement parameters are used.

Background Removal or Shuttering. Anytime a radiographic image is viewed, whether it is film/screen or digital, unexposed borders around the collimation edges allow excess light to enter the eye. Known as *veil glare*, this excess light causes oversensitization of a chemical within the eye called rhodopsin and results in temporary white light blindness. Although the eye recovers quickly enough so that the viewer recognizes only that the light is very bright, it is a great distraction that interferes with image reception by the eye. In film/screen radiography, black cardboard glare masks or special automatic collimation view boxes were sometimes used to lessen the effects of veil glare, but no technique has ever been entirely successful or convenient. In digital imaging, automatic **shuttering** is used to blacken out the white collimation borders, effectively eliminating veil glare. Shuttering is a viewing technique only and should never be used to mask poor collimation practices.

Background removal is also beneficial. Removing the white unexposed borders results in an overall smaller number of pixels and reduces the amount of information to be stored (Figure 3-6).

Image Orientation. **Image orientation** refers to the way anatomy is oriented on the imaging plate. The image reader has to be informed of the location of the patient's head versus the location of the feet and right side versus left side. The image reader scans and reads the image from the leading edge of the imaging plate to the opposite end. The image is displayed exactly as it was read unless the reader is informed differently. Vendors mark the cassettes in different ways to help technologists orient the cassette in such a way that the image will be processed to display as expected. Fuji uses a tape-type orientation marker on the top and right side of the cassette. Kodak uses a sticker reminiscent of the film/screen cassette identification blocker. Some examinations, however, require unusual orientation of the cassette. In these cases, the reader must be informed of the orientation of the anatomy with respect to the reader. With FPD systems, for which no cassette is used, the position of the part should correspond with the marked top and sides of the detector. Refer to the specific manufacturer requirements for part orientation if applicable.

Image Stitching. When anatomy or the area of interest is too large to fit on one cassette, multiple images can be "stitched" together using specialized software programs. This process is called **image stitching**. In some cases special cassette holders are used and positioned vertically, corresponding to foot-to-hip or entire spine studies. Images are processed in computer programs that nearly seamlessly join the anatomy for display as one single image. This technique eliminates the need for large (36-inch) cassettes previously used in film/screen radiography (Figure 3-7).

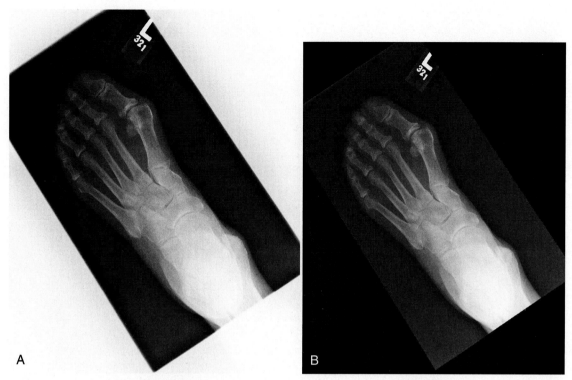

FIGURE 3-6 **Shuttering. A,** AP foot with collimation. **B,** AP foot with collimation and black surround or shuttering. *(Images courtesy Carestream Health, Inc.)*

Image Annotation. Many times, information other than standard identification must be added to the image. In screen/film radiography, time and date stickers, grease pencils, or permanent markers were used to indicate technical factors, time sequences, technologist identification, or position. The **image annotation** function allows selection of preset terms and/or manual text input and can be particularly useful when such additional information is necessary. (Function availability depends on the manufacturer.) The annotations overlay the image as bitmap images. Depending on how each system is set up, annotations may not transfer to the PACS. Again, input of annotation for identification of the patient's left or right side should never be used as a substitute for technologist's anatomy markers (Figure 3-8).

Magnification. Two basic types of magnification techniques come standard with digital systems. One technique functions as a magnifying glass in the sense that a box placed over a small segment of anatomy on the main image shows a magnified version of the underlying anatomy. Both the size of the magnified area and the amount of magnification can be made larger or smaller. The other technique is a zoom technique that allows magnification of the entire image. The image can be enlarged enough so that only parts of it are visible on the screen, but the parts not visible can be reached through mouse navigation (Figure 3-9).

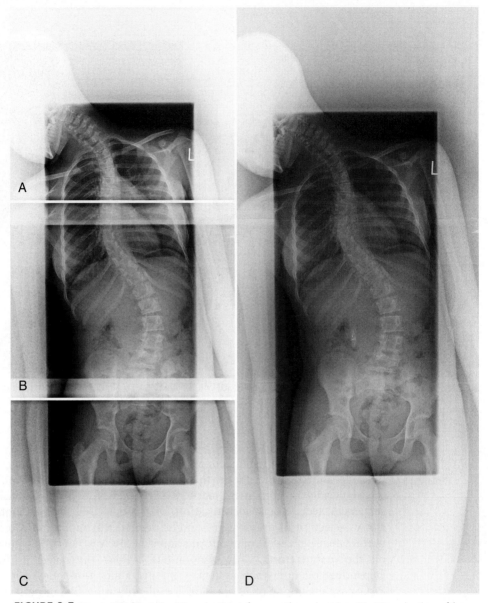

FIGURE 3-7 Image Stitching. A, AP projection of upper thoracic spine. **B,** AP projection of lower thoracic and upper lumbar spine. **C,** AP projection of lower lumbar spine. **D,** All three images joined by digital stitching, resulting in AP projection of entire spine for scoliosis. *(Images courtesy Carestream Health, Inc.)*

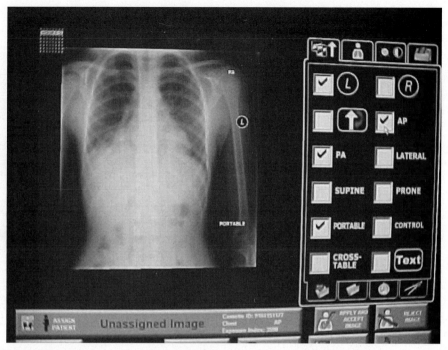

FIGURE 3-8 **Computed Radiography (CR) Workstation Screen for Image Annotation.** Note that even though both PA and AP choices are checked, only the first (PA) shows on the screen.

IMAGE MANAGEMENT

Patient Demographic Input

Proper identification of the patient is even more critical with digital images than with conventional hard copy film/screen images. Retrieval of digital images can be nearly impossible if the images have not been properly and accurately identified. **Patient demographics** include things such as patient name, health care facility, patient identification number, date of birth, and examination date. This information should be input or linked via barcode label scans before the start of the examination and before the processing phase. Occasionally errors are made, and demographic information must be altered. If the technologist performing the examination is absolutely positive that the image is of the correct patient, then demographic information can be altered at the processing stage. This function should be tracked and changes linked to the technologist altering the information to ensure accuracy and accountability.

Problems arise if the patient name is entered differently from visit to visit or examination to examination. For example, if the patient's name is Jane A. Doe and is entered that way, that name must be entered that way for every other examination. If entered as Jane Doe, the system will save it as a different patient. Merging these files can be difficult, especially if there are several versions of the name. If a patient gives a middle name on one visit but has had multiple examinations under

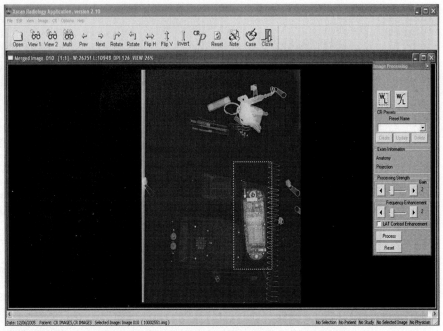

A

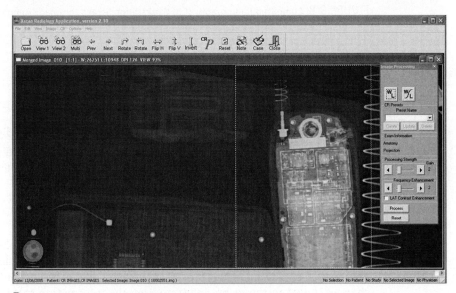

B

FIGURE 3-9 Image Magnification. A, Digital image of various everyday objects. **B,** Magnified view of a cell phone.

his or her first name, retrieval of previous files will be very difficult and in some cases impossible. The right images must be placed in the correct data files just as hard copy films had to be placed in the correct patient folder.

Manual Send

Because the quality control (QC) workstation is networked to the PACS, it also has the capability to send images to local network workstations. The **manual send** function allows the QC technologist to select one or more local computers to receive images.

Archive Query

In the event that the technologist wishes to see historical images, the PACS archive can be queried. **Archive query** is a function that allows retrieval of images from the PACS based on date of examination, patient name or number, examination number, pathologic condition, or anatomic area. For example, the technologist could query or ask the PACS to retrieve all chest x-rays for a particular date or range of dates, or query retrieval of all of a certain patient's images. There are multiple combinations of query fields that can generate reports that include many categories of information or a few very specific categories to be retrieved from storage.

SUMMARY

- Recognition of exposure data involves processing only the optimal density exposure range and generates a graphic representation or histogram of the optimal densities.
- After the plate is scanned and the image location and orientation are determined, a value is placed on each pixel, and the histogram is generated displaying the minimum and maximum diagnostic signal.
- Histograms are different for specific anatomic regions and remain fairly constant from patient to patient.
- Automatic rescaling allows pixel display for the area of interest, regardless of the amount of exposure, unless the exposure is too low or too high. In those cases, quantum mottle or contrast loss occurs.
- There is no substitute for proper kVp and mAs. Insufficient photons, insufficient penetration, or overpenetration results in a loss of diagnostic information that cannot be manufactured by manipulating the image parameters.
- Exposure latitude is slightly greater with digital imaging than with film/screen imaging because of the wider range of exposures recorded with digital systems.
- Contrast enhancement parameters allow enhancement of the image by controlling the steepness of the exposure gradient, density variance, and contrast amount.
- Spatial frequency resolution is controlled by focal spot, OID, and computer algorithms.

- The Nyquist theorem is applied to digital images to ensure sufficient signal sampling for maximum resolution.
- Edge enhancement is accomplished by limiting the number of pixels in a neighborhood of the matrix. Known area-of-interest frequencies can be amplified or high-pass filtered to increase contrast and edge enhancement.
- Suppressing frequencies of lesser importance, known as *masking*, can cause small detail loss.
- Low-pass filtering or smoothing is the result of pixel averaging to remove high-frequency noise. Contrast and noise are decreased, allowing small structures to be seen.
- Window and level parameters control pixel brightness and contrast.
- Shuttering is a process that removes or replaces the background to block distracting light surrounding a digital image. This does not take the place of proper collimation and can be removed to show proper collimation.
- Digital imaging cassettes are marked for orientation to the top and right sides. This ensures that images will be displayed correctly.
- Image stitching is a computer program process that allows multiple images to be joined when the anatomy is too large for one exposure. The result is a nearly seamless single image.
- On digital systems, magnification techniques are available that allow small area enlargement or whole image enlargement.
- Proper patient demographic input is the responsibility of the technologist performing the examination. Any alteration of patient demographics should be avoided unless absolute identification is possible.
- The manual send function allows images to be sent to one or more networked computers.
- Historical study of patient examinations can be accomplished through the archive query function. Querying for retrieval of radiographic studies can be specific to a patient, examination date, or examination type or include a broader search for date ranges, combinations of anatomic areas, and so on.

CHAPTER REVIEW QUESTIONS

1. A graphical representation of a digital image is called a _____.
   a. Matrix
   b. Pixel
   c. Look-up table
   d. Histogram
2. The useful signal is determined during which part of image processing?
   a. Image sampling
   b. Histogram analysis
   c. Exposure indices analysis
   d. Digitization
3. The Nyquist theorem states that the sampling frequency must be less than twice the frequency of the input signal.
   a. True
   b. False

4. Aliasing occurs when the sampling frequency is not greater than twice the frequency of the input signal.
   a. True
   b. False
5. In digital projection radiography, what process is used to normalize an image that has been taken with too great of an exposure?
   a. High-pass filtering
   b. Low-pass filtering
   c. Automatic rescaling
   d. Aliasing
6. The look-up table that is used to determine the brightness and contrast of an image is unique for each anatomic part.
   a. True
   b. False
7. Which processing technique will amplify particular known frequencies in an image while suppressing others?
   a. Edge enhancement
   b. High-pass filtering
   c. Masking
   d. All of the above
8. Window width controls the brightness of the image on the display.
   a. True
   b. False
9. Shuttering the digital image will reduce the exposure to the patient.
   a. True
   b. False
10. Which processing parameter will put together multiple images into one single image for display?
    a. Magnification
    b. Automatic rescaling
    c. Image orientation
    d. Image stitching

PART III

Digital Image
Acquisition

Photostimulable Phosphor Image Capture

Artifacts
    Imaging Plate Artifacts
    Image Processing Artifacts
    Plate Reader Artifacts
    Printer Artifacts
    Operator Errors
Summary

KEY TERMS

Artifacts	Laser
Backing layer	Milliamperage seconds (mAs)
Barcode label	Moiré
Bit depth	Phosphor center
Cassette	Phosphor layer
Color layer	Photodetector
Collimation	Photostimulable phosphor
Conductive layer	Protective layer
Fast scan direction	Reflective layer
Focused grid	Quantum mottle
Grid frequency	Quantum noise
Grid ratio	Shuttering
Imaging plate	Slow scan direction
Kilovoltage peak (kVp)	Support layer

The phrase *digital radiographic image acquisition and processing* is used in this book to categorize the different ways of acquiring and processing digital radiographic images. One way to do this is through photostimulable phosphor (PSP) systems. These systems can be either cassette-based or cassette-less in design. This chapter introduces the process of acquiring an image using PSP technology. Key topics include technical factors, equipment selection, exposure indicators, image data recognition, and artifacts.

The term *radiographic* refers to general x-ray procedures as distinct from other digital modalities such as computed tomography (CT), magnetic resonance imaging (MRI), and ultrasound (US).

This chapter introduces the basic principles of PSP and discusses how PSP equipment works. Some similarities between PSP and conventional radiography are discussed. A basic understanding of how PSP works prepares the technologist to make sound ethical decisions when performing radiographic examinations.

Cassette-based PSP systems differ from conventional radiography in that the cassette is simply a lightproof container that protects an imaging plate from light and handling. The imaging plate takes the place of radiographic film and is capable of storing an image formed by incident x-ray photon excitation of phosphors. The cassette-less systems using PSP technology function in a similar fashion but without the need of a cassette. During the reading process, the phosphor releases the stored light and converts it into an electrical signal, which is then digitized.

Cassette

The PSP **cassette** looks like the conventional screen-film cassette. It consists of a durable, lightweight plastic material (Figure 4-1). The cassette is backed by a thin sheet of aluminum or lead that absorbs backscatter x-ray photons (Figure 4-2). In addition to holding the PSP plate, the cassette contains an antistatic material (usually felt) that protects against static electricity buildup, dust collection, and mechanical damage to the plate (Figure 4-3).

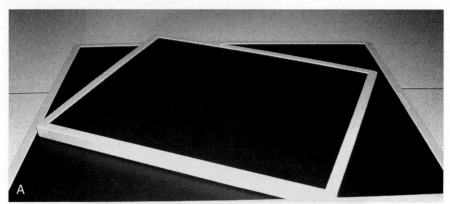

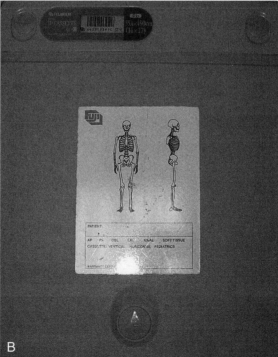

FIGURE 4-1 PSP cassette.

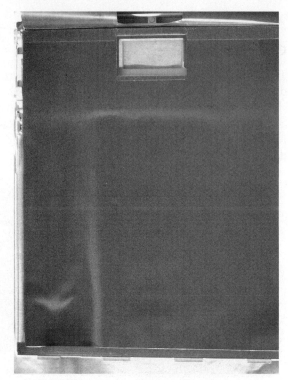

FIGURE 4-2 Aluminum absorber in cassette.

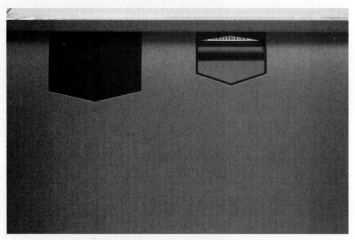

FIGURE 4-3 Antistatic felt in cassette.

Imaging Plate

Construction. In PSP systems, the radiographic image is recorded on a thin sheet of plastic known as the **imaging plate**. The imaging plate consists of several layers (Figure 4-4):

- A **protective layer.** This is a very thin, tough, clear plastic that protects the phosphor layer.
- A **phosphor layer** (or active layer). This is a layer of **photostimulable phosphor** that "traps" electrons during exposure. It is usually made of phosphors from the barium fluorohalide family (e.g., barium fluorohalide, chlorohalide, or bromohalide crystals). This layer may also contain a dye that differentially absorbs the stimulating light to prevent as much spread as possible and functions much the same as dye added to conventional radiographic screens.
- A **reflective layer.** This is a layer that sends light in a forward direction when released in the cassette reader. This layer may be black to reduce the spread of stimulating light and the escape of emitted light. Some detail is lost in this process.
- A **conductive layer.** This is a layer of material that absorbs and reduces static electricity.

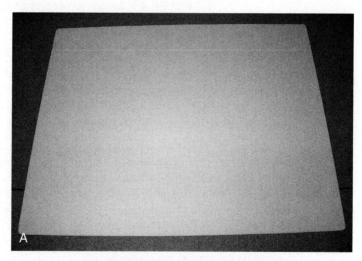

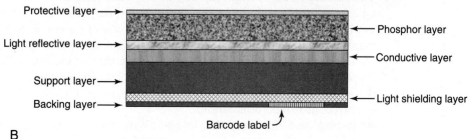

FIGURE 4-4 **A,** Imaging plate. **B,** Construction.

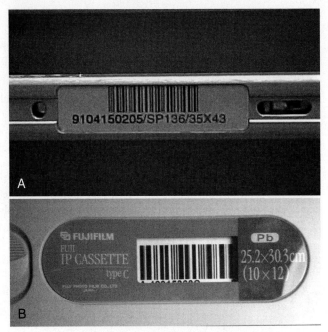

FIGURE 4-5 Barcode identification labels.

- A **color layer**. Newer plates may contain a color layer, located between the active layer and the support, that absorbs the stimulating light but reflects emitted light.
- A **support layer**. This is a semi-rigid material that gives the imaging sheet some strength.
- A **backing layer**. This is a soft polymer that protects the back of the cassette.

Cassette-based PSP systems contain a window with a **barcode label** or barcode sticker on the cassette that allows the technologist to match the image information with the patient-identifying barcode on the examination request (Figure 4-5). For each new examination, the patient-identifying barcode and the barcode label on the cassette must be scanned and connected to the patient position or examination menu. In cassette-less systems, the image must be matched with the examination worklist on the computer and there will not be a paper-type sticker for the plate. The cassette-based system may also have a label such as a colored mark or sticker where applicable to indicate the appropriate orientation of the cassette in relation to the patient (Figure 4-6). When the cassette is oriented correctly, less image manipulation is required after processing. When the examination type is associated with the cassette, an automatic screen orientation of the image is built within the software. If the cassette was correctly oriented, the image will be displayed correctly; if not, the image will need to be rotated or flipped on the screen to display the image in correct anatomic orientation.

Acquiring and Forming the Image. With PSP systems, the patient is x-rayed exactly the same way as in conventional radiography. The patient is positioned using appropriate positioning techniques, and the body part is aligned with the image

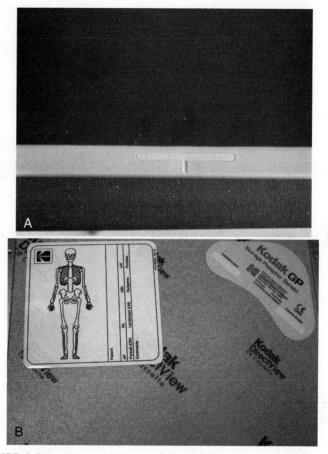

FIGURE 4-6 A, Fuji cassette orientation stickers. **B,** Kodak orientation label.

receptor. The patient is then exposed using the proper combination of kilovoltage peak (kVp), milliamperage seconds (mAs), and distance. The difference lies in how the exposure is recorded. In PSP, the remnant beam interacts with electrons in the barium fluorohalide crystals contained within the imaging plate. This interaction stimulates, or gives energy to, electrons in the crystals, trapping them in an area of the crystal known as the color or **phosphor center**. This trapped signal will remain for hours, even days, although deterioration begins almost immediately. In fact, the trapped signal is never completely lost. That is, a certain amount of an exposure remains trapped so that the imaging plate can never be completely erased. However, the residual trapped electrons are so few in number that they do not interfere with subsequent exposures.

The Reader

There are two types of PSP readers: point scan and line scan. Point scan readers have an optical stage, a scanning laser beam, translation mechanics, a light pickup

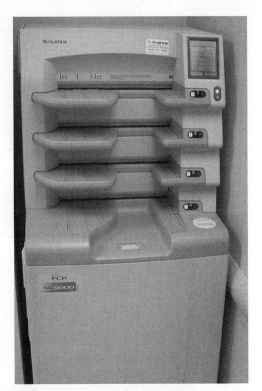

FIGURE 4-7 Fuji SmartPSP PSP reader.

guide, a photomultiplier, a signal transformer/amplifier, and an analog-to-digital converter (ADC). At any point in time, only a single laser point radiates the imaging plate. Line scan readers are based on simultaneous stimulation of the imaging plate one line at a time, and with line scan readers, the acquisition of the photostimulated luminescence (PSL) occurs with a charge-coupled device (CCD) linear array photodetector. PSL refers to the emission of light from the phosphor layer after stimulation by the relevant light source. Instead of a single laser beam, there is a scanning module that contains several linear laser units and optical light collection lenses. The line scan system requires a lens array to focus each laser beam to a corresponding point on the CCD array.

With PSP systems, no chemical processor or darkroom is necessary. Instead, following exposure, the cassette is fed into a reader (Figure 4-7) that removes the imaging plate and scans it with a laser to release the stored electrons. When referring to the PSP interaction within the reader, a technologist often will note two scan directions. **Fast scan direction** is the movement of the laser across the imaging plate (also known as "scan") and **slow scan direction** is the movement of the imaging plate through the reader (also known as "translation" or "sub-scan direction").

The Laser. A laser, or *l*ight *a*mplification of *s*timulated *e*mission of *r*adiation, is a device that creates and amplifies a narrow, intense beam of coherent light (Figure 4-8). The atoms or molecules of a crystal such as ruby or garnet or of a gas, liquid, or other substance are excited so that more of them are at high energy levels rather

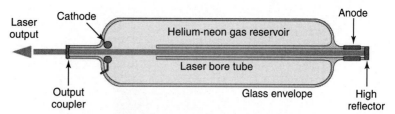

FIGURE 4-8 Laser construction.

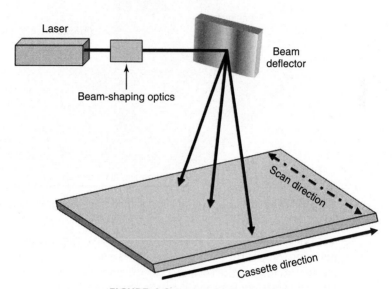

FIGURE 4-9 PSP reader laser optics.

than low energy levels. Surfaces at both ends of the laser container reflect energy back and forth as atoms bombard each other, stimulating the lower energy atoms to emit secondary photons in the same frequency as the bombarding atoms. When the energy builds sufficiently, the atoms discharge simultaneously as a burst of coherent light; it is coherent because all of the photons are traveling in the same direction at the same frequency. The laser requires a constant power source to prevent output fluctuations. The laser beam passes through beam-shaping optics to an optical mirror that directs the laser beam to the surface of the imaging plate (Figure 4-9).

Using the Laser to Read the Imaging Plate. During the reading process, the imaging plate is scanned with a helium laser beam or, in more recent systems, solid-state laser diodes. This beam, about 100 micrometers (μm) wide with a wavelength of 633 nanometers (nm) (or 670 to 690 nm for solid state), scans the plate with red light in a raster pattern and gives energy to the trapped electrons. The red laser light is emitted at approximately 2 electron volts eV, which is necessary to energize the trapped electrons. This extra energy allows the trapped electrons to escape the active layer where they emit visible blue light at an energy of 3 eV as they relax into lower energy levels (Figure 4-10). As the imaging plate moves through or remains

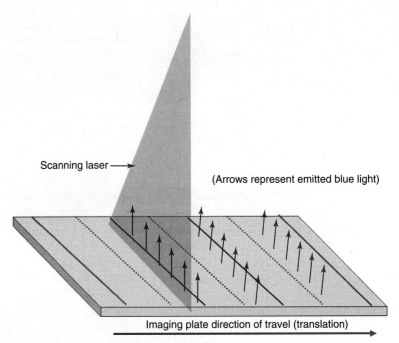

Scanning laser ⟶

(Arrows represent emitted blue light)

Imaging plate direction of travel (translation) ⟶

FIGURE 4-10 The laser scans the imaging plate, releasing stored energy as blue light (*arrows*).

stationary in the reader, the laser scans across the imaging plate multiple times. The plate movement through the scanner is known as translation because it moves in a parallel manner at a certain rate through the reader. This scan process produces lines of light intensity information that are detected by a photodetector. The **photodetector** amplifies the light and sends it to an ADC. The translation speed of the plate must be coordinated with the scan direction of the laser, or the spacing of the scan lines will be affected.

The action of moving the laser beam across the imaging plate is much like holding a flashlight at the same height and moving it back and forth across a wall. The more angled the beam is, the more elliptical the shape of the beam. The same thing happens with the reader laser beam as it scans. This means that if this change in the beam shape were ignored, the output of the screen would differ from the middle to the edges, resulting in differing spatial resolution and inconsistent output signals, depending on the position and angle of the laser beam. To correct this, the beam is "shaped" by special optics that keep the beam size, shape, and speed largely independent of the beam position. A beam deflector moves the laser beam rapidly back and forth across the imaging plate to stimulate the phosphors. Mirrors are used to ensure that the beam is positioned consistently. Because the type of phosphor material in the imaging plate has an effect on the amount of energy required, the laser and the imaging plate should be designed to work together. The light collection optics direct the released phosphor energy to an optical filter and then to the photodetector (Figure 4-11).

Although there will be variances among manufacturers, the typical throughput is 50 cassettes per hour. Some manufacturers claim that a rate of up to 150 cassettes

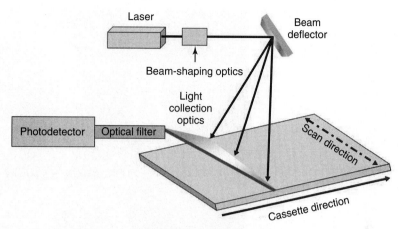

FIGURE 4-11 Laser optics.

per hour is possible, but based on average hospital department work flow, 50 cassettes per hour is a more realistic expectation.

Digitizing the Signal. When we talk about digitizing a signal, such as the light signal from a photodetector, we are talking about assigning a numerical value to each light photon. As humans, we experience the world analogically. We see the world as infinitely smooth gradients of shape and color. *Analog* refers to a device or system that represents changing values as continuously variable physical quantities. A typical analog device is a watch: the hands move continuously around the face and are capable of indicating every possible time of day. In contrast, a digital clock is capable of representing only a finite number of times (e.g., every tenth of a second). The scanning process results in the conversion of the light emitted from the storage phosphor into an electrical signal. The electrical signal is sampled and digitized to represent a specific location within the image matrix and displays as a specific brightness. A matrix is the group of squares that make up the image information.

Each square is called a *pixel* or *picture element*. The typical number of pixels in a matrix ranges from about 512×512 to 1024×1024 for CT but can be as large as 2500×2500 for radiography. The more pixels there are, the greater the image resolution for a fixed field of view. The image is digitized both by position (spatial location) and by intensity (gray level). Each pixel contains bits of information, and the number of bits per pixel that define the shade of each pixel is known as **bit depth**. If a pixel has a bit depth of 8, for example, then the number of gray tones that pixel can produce is 2 to the power of the bit depth, or 2^8, or 256 shades of gray. Therefore the number of photons detected within the pixel will determine the amount of gray level or bit depth within that pixel. Some PSP systems have bit depths of 10 or 12, resulting in more shades of gray. Each pixel can have a gray level between 1 (2^0) and 4096 (2^{20}). The gray level will be a factor in determining the quality of the image.

Spatial Resolution. The amount of detail present in any image is known as its *spatial resolution.* Just as the crystal size and thickness of the phosphor layer determine resolution in film/screen radiography, phosphor layer thickness and pixel size

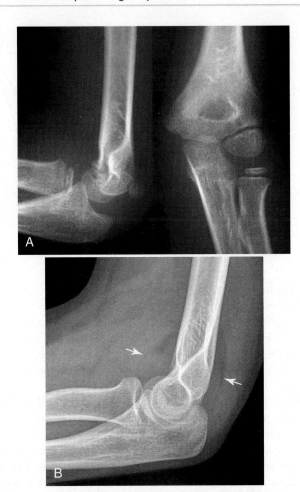

FIGURE 4-12 A, Film/screen elbow radiograph. **B,** PSP elbow image. Note the ability to better visualize the fat pads on the lateral view. (**A** *courtesy Dr. Loren Yamamoto. Appeared in Inaba, AS. Radiographic examination of the elbow: The hourglass sign. In:* Radiology cases in emergency medicine. *Vol. 1.)*

help determine resolution in PSP. The thinner the phosphor layer, the higher the resolution. In film/screen radiography, resolution at its best is limited to approximately 10 line pairs (lp) per millimeter (mm). In general projection radiography PSP imaging, resolution is approximately 2.55 to 5 lp/mm, resulting in less detail. Resolution detail is also affected by the laser beam spot size, translation speed, sampling frequency, and the laser beam sweep in point beam readers. However, because the bit depth, or the number of available shades of gray that can be displayed, is much higher, the difference in resolution is more difficult to discern. More tissue densities on the digital radiograph are seen, giving the appearance of more detail. For example, the fat pads on a lateral elbow are difficult to discern on a film image (Figure 4-12A). Fat pads are a very important sign for the radiologists to see in

Strong light source

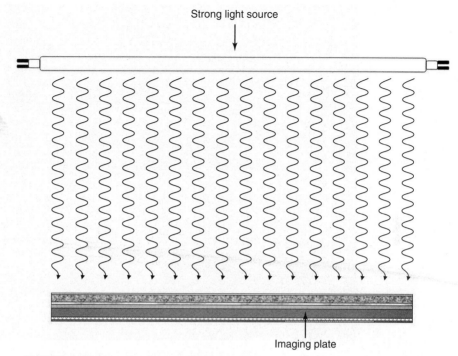

Imaging plate

FIGURE 4-13 Fluorescent floodlight is used to remove any remaining trapped energy.

pediatric elbow fractures. In the digital image, the fat pads are easily seen (Figure 4-12B). This is because of the ability to display more shades of gray, thereby making it possible to visualize more tissues of varying densities; this does not, however, mean that the digital image contains additional detail.

Erasing the Image. The process of reading the image returns most but not all of the electrons to a lower energy state, effectively removing the image from the plate. However, imaging plates are extremely sensitive to scatter radiation and should be erased to prevent a buildup of background signal. At least once a week the plates should be run under an erase cycle to remove background radiation and scatter. PSP readers have an erasure mode that allows the surface of the imaging plate to be scanned without recoding the generated signal. Systems automatically erase the plate by flooding it with light to remove any electrons still trapped after the initial plate reading (Figure 4-13). Cassettes should be erased before using if the last time of erasure is unknown.

Preprocessing, Processing, and Forwarding the Image. Once the imaging plate has been read, the signal is sent to the computer where it is preprocessed. The data then go to a monitor where the technologist can review the image, manipulate it if necessary (postprocessing), and send it to the quality control (QC) station and ultimately to the picture archiving and communication system (PACS).

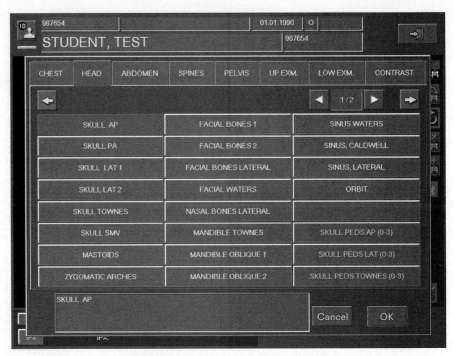

FIGURE 4-14 Workstation menu skull selection.

EXPOSURE

Part Selection

Depending on the type of system being used, the technologist will choose the body part imaged either prior to exposure of the image receptor or after exposure. If the examination room has a PSP housed in the detector in the table or a wall stand, the patient worklist will most likely be in the room's workstation, which means the technologist may choose the appropriate body part automatically. Always check to make sure the appropriate part has been selected. When using a cassette-based system, the selection of the body part is usually done after exposure and it is imperative that cassettes are kept apart so that the technologist knows which cassette goes with which body part. For example, if a skull examination is to be performed, the technologist would choose "skull" from the workstation menu (Figure 4-14). Selecting the proper body part and position is important for the proper conversion to take place. Image recognition is accomplished through complex mathematical computer algorithms, and if the improper part and/or position is designated, the image may be processed incorrectly and fail to display properly. For example, if a knee examination is to be performed and the examination selected is for skull, the computer will interpret the exposure for the skull, resulting in improper image display (Figure 4-15). The resultant image might appear too dark or too light and it might appear grainy or like it was underexposed. It is not acceptable to select a body part

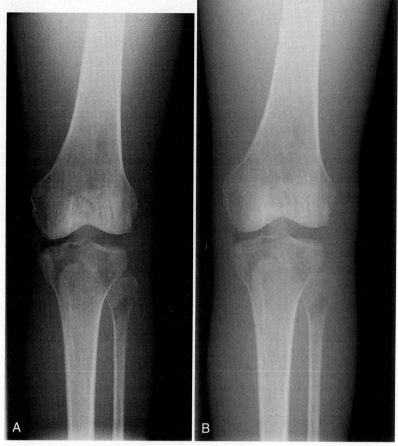

FIGURE 4-15 A, Anteroposterior (AP) knee with proper menu selection. **B,** AP knee with AP skull selected.

or position other than that being performed simply because it provides a better image. If the proper examination/part selection results in a suboptimal image, then service personnel should be notified of the problem to correct it as soon as possible. Improper menu selections may lead to overexposure of the patient and/or repeated exposure.

Technical Factors

Kilovoltage Peak Selection. Kilovoltage peak (kVp), milliamperage seconds (mAs), and distance are chosen in exactly the same manner in digital projection systems as in conventional film/screen radiography. Traditionally, kVp was chosen for penetration and tissue type and mAs according to the number of photons required for that body part. kVp values range from 45 to 120 on most digital projection systems. It is not recommended that kVp values lower than 45 or greater than 120 be used because those values may be inconsistent and produce too little

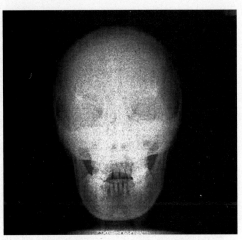

FIGURE 4-16 Grainy appearance because of insufficient light produced in imaging plate.

or too much excitation of the phosphors. The k-edge of phosphor imaging plates ranges from 30 to 50 kiloelectron volt (keV) so that exposure ranges of 60 to 110 kVp are optimum. However, exposures outside that range are widely used and will depend on the image quality desired. Remember, the process of attenuation of the x-ray beam is exactly the same as in conventional film/screen radiography. It takes the same kVp to penetrate the abdomen with PSP systems as it did with a film/screen system. It is vital that the proper balance between patient dose and part penetration be achieved. A major difference between film/screen and digital receptors is that digital image contrast is no longer dependent on kVp. Sufficient kVp is needed to penetrate the body part; however, higher kVp values can be used, allowing for lower mAs values. The dynamic recording range of digital receptors is much higher than those used in film/screen systems and inherently produces a wide variety of gray values. Contrast is determined by computer processing.

Milliamperage Seconds Selection. Again, the mAs is selected according to the number of photons needed for a particular part. If there are too few photons, no matter what level of kVp is chosen, the result will be a lack of sufficient phosphor stimulation. When insufficient light is produced, the image is grainy, a condition known as **quantum mottle** or **quantum noise** (Figure 4-16). PSP systems typically use automatic exposure controls (AECs), just as many film/screen systems do. When converting from film/screen systems to a PSP system, it is critical that the AECs be recalibrated to the desired exposure indicator.

Equipment Selection

Imaging Plate Selection. Two important factors should be considered when selecting the PSP imaging cassette: type and size. Most manufacturers produce two types of imaging plates: standard and high resolution. Cassettes should be marked on the outside to indicate high-resolution imaging plates. High-resolution imaging plates contain a thinner phosphor layer as compared to the standard plates. The thinner

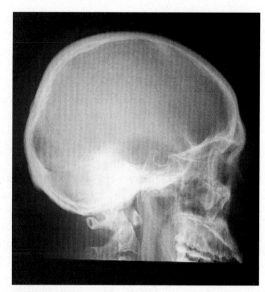

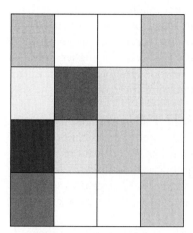

FIGURE 4-17 Pixel matrix.

FIGURE 4-18 Lateral skull image displaying moiré pattern artifact caused by incorrect grid alignment with laser scan direction.

layer results in greater image sharpness because of the reduced amount of light spreading in more lateral directions. When light spreads laterally, it causes the images to appear somewhat blurry. This occurs with any image capture system that involves the release of light. Typically, high-resolution imaging plates are limited to the smaller cassette sizes and are most often used for extremities, mammography, and other examinations requiring increased detail.

PSP digital images are displayed in a matrix of pixels (Figure 4-17), and the pixel size is an important factor in determining the resolution of the displayed image. As a review from Chapter 2, if the matrix of an imaging system remains constant, as the field of view decreases, the pixel size also decreases and the spatial resolution of the image increases. Therefore the technologist should use the smallest field appropriate for the body part being imaged so that the pixel size will be at its smallest and the spatial resolution will be at its highest. Appropriate image plate selection for the examination also eliminates scatter outside the initial collimation by reducing the amount of imaging plate not being exposed, and this increases contrast resolution.

Grid Selection. Digital images are displayed in tiny rows of picture elements or pixels. Grid lines that are projected onto the imaging plate when using a stationary grid can interfere with the image. This results in a wavy artifact known as a **moiré** pattern that occurs because the grid lines and the scanning laser are parallel (Figure 4-18). The oscillating motion of a moving grid, or Bucky, blurs the grid lines and eliminates the interference. Because the PSP systems are more sensitive to low levels of radiation, the use of a grid is much more critical than in film/screen radiography. Appropriate selection of stationary grids reduces this interference as well. Grid selection factors are frequency, ratio, and focus.

Frequency. **Grid frequency** refers to the number of grid lines per centimeter or lines per inch. The higher the frequency or the more lines per inch, the finer the grid lines in the image and the less they interfere with the image. Typical grid frequency is between 80 and 152 lines/inch. Some manufacturers recommend no fewer than 103 lines/inch and strongly suggest grid frequencies greater than 150. The higher frequency grids require more x-ray photons to produce an image than lower frequency grids require, therefore the patient will receive a higher dose. In addition, the closer the grid frequency is to the laser scanning frequency, the greater likelihood of frequency harmonics or matching and the more likely the risk of moiré effects.

Ratio. The relationship between the height of the lead strips and the space between the lead strips is known as **grid ratio.** The higher the ratio, the more scatter radiation is absorbed. However, the higher the ratio, the more critical the positioning is, so high grid ratio is not a good choice for mobile radiography. A grid ratio of 6:1 would be proper for mobile radiography, whereas a 12:1 grid ratio would be appropriate for departmental grids that are more stable and less likely to be mispositioned, causing grid cutoff errors.

Focus. Most grids chosen by radiography departments are parallel and focused. Parallel grids are less critical to beam centering but should not be used at distances less than 48 inches. **Focused grids** consist of lead strips angled to coincide with the divergence of the x-ray beam and must be used within specific distances using a precisely centered beam.

Collimation

When exposing a patient, the larger the volume of tissue being irradiated, the more scatter will be produced. Whereas the use of a grid absorbs the scatter that exits the patient and affects latent image formation, properly used collimation reduces the area of irradiation and the volume of tissue in which scatter can be created. **Collimation** is the reduction of the area of beam that reaches the patient through the use of two pairs of lead shutters encased in a housing attached to the x-ray tube. Collimation results in increased contrast resolution as a result of the reduction of scatter. Through postexposure image manipulation known as **shuttering**, a black background can be added around the original collimation edges, virtually eliminating the distracting white or clear areas (Figure 4-19). However, this technique is not a replacement for proper preexposure collimation. It is an image aesthetic only and does not change the amount or angles of scatter. There is no substitute for appropriate collimation because collimation reduces patient dose.

Side/Position Markers

Anyone who has used digital image processing equipment knows that it is very easy to mark images with left and right side markers or other position or text markers after the exposure has been made. However, we strongly advise that conventional lead markers be used the same way they are used in film/screen systems. Marking the patient examination at the time of exposure not only identifies the patient's side but also identifies the technologist performing the examination. This is also an issue

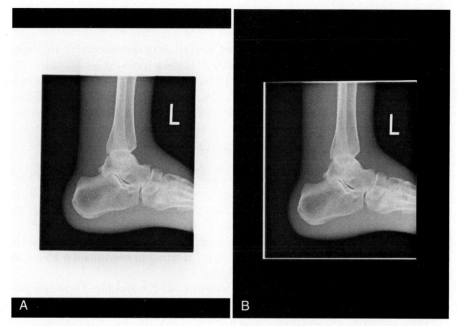

FIGURE 4-19 **A,** Lateral ankle without shuttering. **B,** Lateral ankle with shuttering.

of legality. If the examination results are used in a court case, the images that include the technologist's markers allow the possibility of technologist testimony and lend credibility to his or her expertise.

When all of the appropriate technical factors and equipment have been selected, the image receptor may be exposed and then subjected to the reading process. The image will then be displayed. The radiographer must then consider a number of factors: image exposure indicators, image processing modes, and image processing parameters.

Image Data Recognition and Preprocessing

The image recognition phase is extremely important in establishing the parameters that determine collimation borders and edges, and histogram formation. A histogram is a graphic representation of the numerical tone values of an x-ray exposure. All PSP systems have image recognition, and each has a specific name for this process. Agfa uses the term *collimation*, Carestream uses the term *segmentation*, and Fuji uses the phrase *exposure data recognition*. All systems use a region of interest to define the area where the part to be examined is recognized, and the exposure outside the region of interest is subtracted. Each vendor has a specific tool for different situations such as neck, breasts, pediatrics, and hips in which the anatomy requires some special recognition. Please refer to each vendor's manual to learn their proprietary recognition and processing parameters. The science behind each of these is beyond the scope of this book.

ARTIFACTS

As with film/screen systems, artifacts can degrade images in digital systems. **Artifacts** are any undesirable densities on the processed image other than those caused by scatter radiation or fog. There are four common types of artifacts (in addition to operator errors that may cause artifacts): imaging plate artifacts, plate reader artifacts, image processing artifacts, and printer artifacts.

Imaging Plate Artifacts

As the imaging plate ages, it becomes prone to cracks from the action of removing and replacing the imaging plate within the reader. Cracks in the imaging plate appear as areas of radiolucency on the image (Figure 4-20). The imaging plate must be replaced when cracks occur in clinically useful areas. Adhesive tape used to secure lead markers to a surface can leave residue behind (Figure 4-21). If static exists because of low humidity, hair can cling to the imaging plate, creating another type of image plate artifact (Figure 4-22).

Backscatter created by x-ray photons transmitted through the back of the cassette can cause dark line artifacts (Figure 4-23). Areas of the lead coating on the cassette that are worn or cracked allow scatter to image these weak areas. Proper collimation and regular cassette inspection help to eliminate this problem.

Image Processing Artifacts

Processing artifacts can occur for many different reasons, such as choosing the incorrect processing parameter for a particular part or incorrect sampling of the image file. As discussed previously, it is very important to set appropriate technical factors and choose the correct body part so that the software algorithms will produce the desired image. Poor technique (collimation, grid selection, mAs, kVp, etc.) and positioning can cause these algorithms to misrepresent the image. The technologist must remain aware of all factors that can influence change in the final processed image.

Plate Reader Artifacts

The intermittent appearance of extraneous line patterns can be caused by problems in the plate reader's electronics (Figure 4-24). Reader electronics may have to be replaced to remedy this problem.

White lines that are parallel to the direction of plate travel are caused by dirt, dust, or scratches on the light guide. Service personnel will need to clean or replace the light guide.

A rare but possible artifact can occur when multiple imaging plates are loaded into a single cassette. In this instance, usually only one of the plates will be extracted, which leaves the other plate to be exposed multiple times. The result is similar to a conventional film/screen double-exposed cassette (Figure 4-25).

Insufficient erasure after an overexposure may result in residual image information being left in the imaging plate before the next exposure. This may also occur

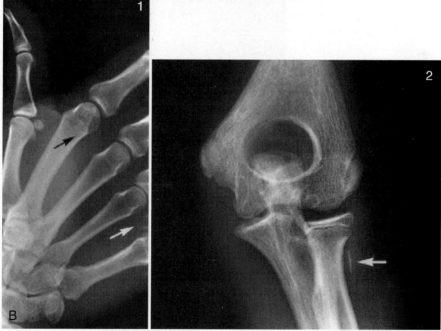

FIGURE 4-20 A, Cracks in the imaging plate which produce areas of radiolucency. **B,** Imaging plate (IP) artifact. (1) Thumb radiograph showing cracks (*white arrow*) that usually first become visible on the IP edges. As deterioration progresses, cracks appear closer to the clinically used areas of the IP (*black arrow*). (2) In some instances, early cracking along the edge of the IP does not occur. This crack appears as a lucency near the radius, which could be confused with a foreign body. (***B*** *Reproduced with permission from Cesar LJ, Schueler BA, Zink FE, et al. Br J Radiol 2001;74:195-202.*)

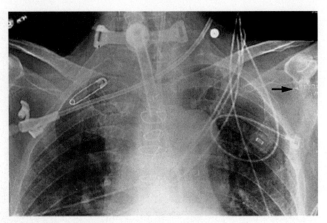

FIGURE 4-21 Residue from adhesive tape used to attach lead markers to the outside of the cassette has caused artifacts *(arrow)* when the tape came in contact with the imaging plate. *(Reproduced with permission from Cesar LJ, Schueler BA, Zink FE, et al. Br J Radiol 2001;74:195-202.)*

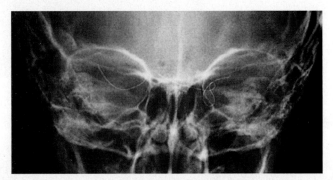

FIGURE 4-22 Static caused a hair to cling to the imaging plate (IP) on this skull image. *(Reproduced with permission from Cesar LJ, Schueler BA, Zink FE, et al. Br J Radiol 2001;74:195-202.)*

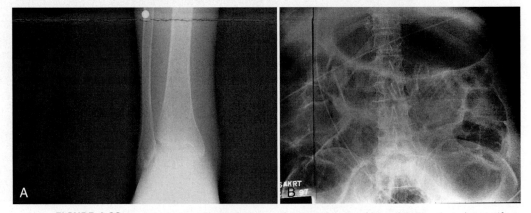

FIGURE 4-23 Backscatter causing dark line artifacts on **A,** AP ankle and **B,** imaging plate artifact. The dark line along the lateral portion of this upper abdomen is caused by backscatter transmitted through the back of the cassette. The line corresponds to the cassette hinge where the lead coating was weakened or cracked. Artifact remedy: to reduce backscatter, the radiographer should collimate when possible. Since backscatter cannot be eliminated in every case, knowledge of the radiographic appearance of cassette backs is useful. *(Reproduced with permission from Cesar LJ, Schueler BA, Zink FE, et al. Br J Radiol 2001,74:195-202.)*

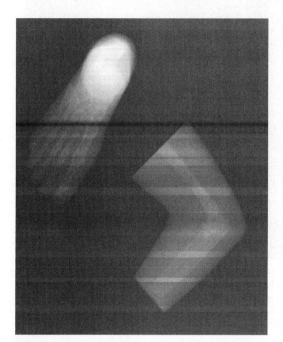

FIGURE 4-24 Extraneous line patterns caused by noise in the plate reader electronics. *(Courtesy Carestream Health, Inc.)*

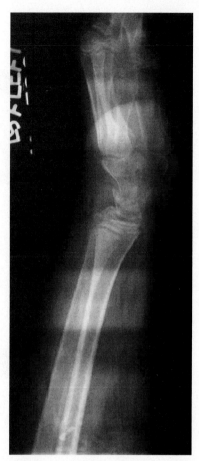

FIGURE 4-25 This artifact occurred because the plate reader loaded two imaging plates (IPs) in a single cassette. After an exposure, the bottom IP was extracted, read, and replaced as usual, leaving the top IP to be exposed numerous times. Artifact remedy: double-loaded cassettes will be discovered during routine IP cleaning. If a cassette containing two IPs is discovered, the IPs should be erased before being put back into use. *(Reproduced with permission from Cesar LJ, Schueler BA, Zink FE, et al. Br J Radiol 2001;74:195-202.)*

if the erasure lamp is in need of repair. The results will vary depending on how much residual image is left and where it is located.

The orientation of a stationary grid relative to the direction of the laser scan is critical to reduce the likelihood of the moiré artifact (Figure 4-26). The grid lines must be perpendicular to the laser scan direction. Moving grids generally do not demonstrate the moiré artifact because the grid lines are blurred out. Vendors have identified the specific grid frequency for stationary grids that will prevent the moiré artifact with their equipment.

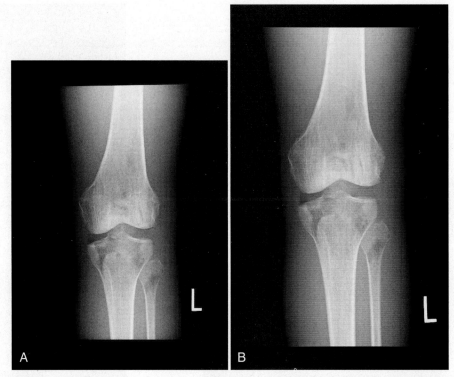

FIGURE 4-26 A, An exposure of a correctly oriented grid with the grid lines perpendicular to the plate reader's scan lines. **B,** A moiré pattern caused by an incorrectly oriented grid, with the grid lines parallel to the plate reader's scan lines.

Printer Artifacts

Fine white lines may appear on the image because of debris on the mirror in the laser printer. Service personnel will need to clean the printer.

Operator Errors

Insufficient collimation can result in an improper calculation of the exposure indicator. This may result in a misrepresentation of the displayed image (Figure 4-27).

If the cassette is exposed with the back of a cassette toward the source, the result will be artifacts from any hinges or other hardware present on the back of the cassettes. Care should be taken to expose only the tube side of the cassette (Figure 4-28).

Underexposure produces quantum mottle, and overexposure reduces contrast. The proper selection of technical factors is critical for both patient dose, image quality, and to ensure the appropriate production of light from the imaging plate (Figure 4-29).

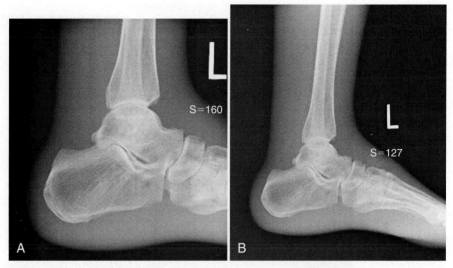

FIGURE 4-27 Insufficient Collimation Error. A, Properly collimated lateral ankle. **B,** Improper collimation resulting in poor histogram analysis. Note the differences in contrast and exposure indices.

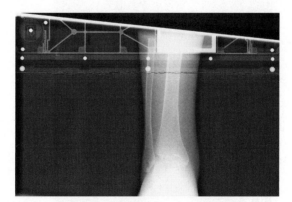

FIGURE 4-28 This AP ankle was exposed through the back of a cassette. Artifact remedy: be sure radiographers are well educated about how to use the entire computed radiography system.

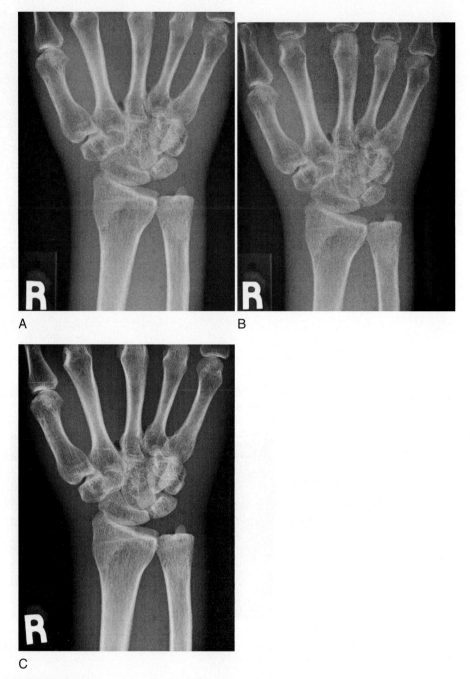

FIGURE 4-29 A, Optimal image. **B,** Underexposed image caused by insufficient mAs, resulting in quantum mottle (best demonstrated in soft tissue between metacarpals) (high kVp, low mAs). **C,** Overexposed image caused by insufficient kVp, resulting in contrast loss (low kVp, high mAs).

SUMMARY

- A PSP cassette-based imaging system has a specially designed cassette made of durable, lightweight plastic.
- The imaging plate is multilayered with protective, phosphor, reflective, conductive, color, support, and backing layers.
- Barcodes are used to identify the cassette or imaging plate and examination request to link the imaging plate with the patient examination.
- Barium fluorohalide crystals in the imaging plate release light energy, which is then stored in the conductive layer.
- The imaging plate reader uses a laser or a module of lasers to scan the imaging plate, releasing the energy stored in the active layer as blue light.
- A photodetector collects the light and sends it to a signal digitizer.
- The analog-to-digital convertor (ADC) assigns a numerical value to each pixel in a matrix according to the intensity of the detected light.
- Spatial resolution of the digital image is determined by the thickness of the phosphor layer and the size of the pixels. The thinner the phosphor layer, the greater the sharpness of the image, and the smaller the pixel size, the higher the spatial resolution.
- The contrast resolution of a digital projection imaging system is higher because the bit depth, or the number of available shades of gray that can be displayed, is higher than in conventional film/screen systems. Because energy stored in the imaging plate dissipates over time, imaging plates should be read as quickly as possible to avoid losing image information.
- Images are sent to the QC station where they are analyzed and sent to the PACS for long-term storage.
- Imaging plates are erased by exposing them to bright light such as fluorescent light.

CHAPTER REVIEW QUESTIONS

1. The active layer in a PSP plate is usually made of phosphors from what family group?
   a. Barium sulfate
   b. Barium fluorohalide
   c. Cesium iodide
   d. Amorphous selenium
2. Which layer of the PSP plate sends light in a more forward direction when released in the reader?
   a. Reflective
   b. Conductive
   c. Phosphor
   d. Support

3. Which layer of the PSP plate reduces static electricity?
   a. Reflective
   b. Conductive
   c. Phosphor
   d. Felt material
4. The barcode label is used by the reader to identify the PSP plate.
   a. True
   b. False
5. The laser excites the electrons trapped in the phosphor centers so that the energy may be released in the form of _____.
   a. Electrons
   b. X-rays
   c. Light
   d. All of the above
6. What device in the reader detects the light being released from the PSP plate during reading?
   a. Laser
   b. Photodetector
   c. Analog-to-digital converter (ADC)
   d. Mirror optics
7. The PSP plate is erased:
   a. After every PSP plate is read.
   b. By flooding it with bright light.
   c. Manually by selecting the proper eraser method.
   d. All of the above
8. Too much mAs will cause quantum mottle.
   a. True
   b. False
9. If grid lines are present and run parallel to the scanning laser, the image will not have the moiré pattern present.
   a. True
   b. False
10. Overexposure will reduce the contrast resolution of the image.
    a. True
    b. False

TFT Flat-Panel Array Image Acquisition

OBJECTIVES

On completion of this chapter, you should be able to:
- Define a thin-film transistor (TFT) flat-panel digital image detector.
- Describe the construction of direct and indirect TFT flat-panel detector systems.
- Differentiate between direct and indirect image capture.
- Describe a gadolinium oxysulphide (Gd_2O_2S) detector.
- Describe a thallium doped cesium iodide (CsI[TI]) detector.
- Relate the design of a TFT flat-panel detector to its performance measurements.
- Describe the cause of image lag and the process of correcting.

OUTLINE

KEY TERMS

Active-matrix flat-panel imagers (AMFPI)

Direct conversion

Field effect transistor (FET)

Flat-panel detector

Gadolinium oxysulphide (Gd_2O_2S)

Gain calibration

Hydrogenated amorphous silicon (a-Si:H)

Image artifacts

Image lag

Indirect conversion

Offset correction

Photoconductors

Sensing component

Switching component

Thallium doped cesium iodide (CsI[TI])

Thin-film transistor (TFT)

The first **thin-film transistor (TFT)** flat-panel amorphous silicon and amorphous selenium detectors were introduced in 1995. These were the first devices to move beyond the cassette into detectors that would reside in the table and wall stand. Today these detectors are no longer permanent fixtures in these two pieces of equipment but can be used portably as a wireless device. With **flat-panel detectors,** the materials used for detecting the x-ray signal and the sensors for recognizing that signal are permanently enclosed inside a rigid protective housing. This chapter will explore these devices and differentiate between the two major types of x-ray signal conversion: indirect and direct.

ACTIVE-MATRIX FLAT-PANEL IMAGERS

Active-matrix flat-panel imagers (AMFPI) consist of a flat-panel array with an x-ray absorption material. The two main types of x-ray absorption materials currently being used are photoconductors and scintillators. **Photoconductors** are materials that absorb x-rays, resulting in an electrical charge. Scintillators are phosphors that produce light when absorbing x-rays. An AMFPI detector measures the response of these materials to x-ray absorption and is a large area two-dimensional (2-D) array of pixels fastened to a thin glass backing, or substrate. The absorption material is attached to the surface of this array either electrically, as in the case of the photoconductor, or physically, as in the case of the phosphor material. The 2-D array functions as a very efficient device that measures x-ray absorption rather than counting or measuring the actual x-rays. The choice of x-ray absorption material determines whether the detector is direct conversion or indirect conversion.

Direct Conversion

In **direct conversion,** x-ray photons are absorbed by the coating material and immediately converted into an electrical signal. The flat-panel detector has a radiation-conversion material or photoconductor, typically made of amorphous selenium

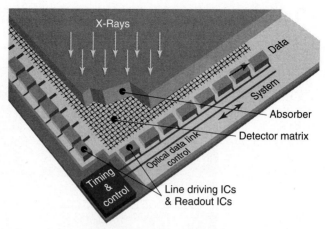

FIGURE 5-1 Flat-Panel Detector Showing the Recording Process. Integrated Circuits, *ICs*.

(a-Se) that is about 500 μm thick for radiography and 200 to 250 μm thick for mammography. This material absorbs x-rays and converts them to electrons, which are stored in the TFT detectors (Figure 5-1). The TFT is a photosensitive array made up of small (about 100 to 200 μm) pixels, also called a detector element (del) in these TFT arrays. Each pixel contains a photodiode that absorbs the electrons and generates electrical charges. A **field effect transistor (FET)** or silicon TFT isolates each pixel element and reacts like a switch to send the electrical charges to the image processor (Figure 5-2). More than 1 million pixels can be read and converted to a composite digital image in less than 1 second. A line of TFT switches, each associated with a storage capacitor, allows the electrical charge information to discharge when the switches are closed. The information is discharged onto the data columns and read out with dedicated electronics. Specialized silicon integrated circuits are connected along the edges of the detector matrix. On one side, integrated circuits control the line scanning sequence, and on the other side, low-noise, high-sensitivity amplifiers perform the readout, amplification, and analog-to-digital conversion. High-speed digital electronics are then used to achieve fast image acquisition and processing.

Indirect Conversion

Indirect-conversion detectors are similar to direct detectors in that they use TFT technology. Unlike direct conversion, **indirect conversion** is a two-step process: x-ray photons are converted to light, and then the light photons are converted to an electrical signal. A phosphor such as gadolinium oxysulphide (Gd_2O_2S), or **thallium doped cesium iodide (CsI[TI])** rapidly absorbs x-rays and produces light. The phosphor layer is known as the scintillation layer. The scintillation layer can be either structured or unstructured. Unstructured layers produce more scattered light than structured layers, thereby decreasing the efficiency of the detector. The light is then

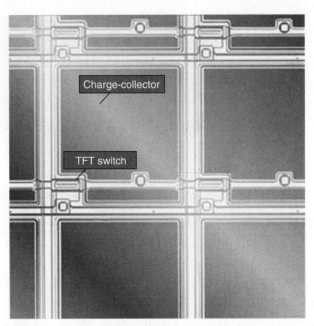

FIGURE 5-2 Anatomy of an Indirect Flat-Panel Detector. *TFT*, Thin-Film Transistor.

converted into an electric charge by a photodetector such as a **hydrogenated amorphous silicon (a-Si:H)** photodiode array. The two-step process occurs as follows:

Step 1: X-ray photons striking the dielectric receptor are absorbed by a scintillation or phosphor material in the imaging plate that converts the incident x-ray photon energy to light.

Step 2: A photosensitive array, made up of small (about 100 to 200 μm) pixels, converts the light into electrical charges. Each pixel contains a photodiode that absorbs the light from the scintillator and generates electrical charges. A FET or silicon TFT isolates each pixel element and reacts like a switch to send the electrical charges to the image processor. As with direct conversion, more than 1 million pixels can be read and converted to a composite digital image in less than 1 second (Figure 5-3).

Gd_2O_2S Detectors. The **gadolinium oxysulphide (Gd_2O_2S)** detecting material is made from small crystals bound together in an unstructured or turbid (powdered granules) layer along with a polyurethane material. The crystalline layer is filled with air pockets that allow light that was generated in the phosphor to escape. It also allows light to escape laterally before it reaches the surface, reducing the efficiency of the phosphor and lowering spatial resolution (Figure 5-4). Gd_2O_2S was used primarily for applications that required a rugged detector, such as portable detectors either wired or wireless. The ruggedness was a result of the unstructured or phosphor layer.

CsI Detectors. The most popular type of amorphous silicon detector uses a CsI scintillator. The scintillator is made by growing very thin crystalline needles (5 to 10 μm wide) perpendicular to the detector surface; these crystalline needles work

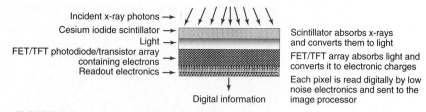

Incident x-ray photons →
Cesium iodide scintillator →
Light →
FET/TFT photodiode/transistor array
containing electrons →
Readout electronics →

Scintillator absorbs x-rays
and converts them to light

FET/TFT array absorbs light and
converts it to electronic charges

Each pixel is read digitally by low
noise electronics and sent to the
image processor

Digital information

FIGURE 5-3 Thin-Film Transistor. *FET*, field effect transistor; *TFT*, thin-film transistor.

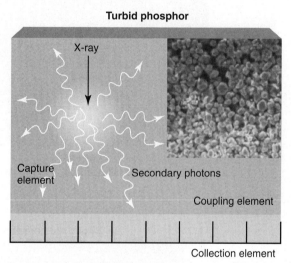

Turbid phosphor

X-ray

Capture
element

Secondary photons

Coupling element

Collection element

FIGURE 5-4 Gadolinium Oxysulphide Scintillator Showing Light Spread Potential. *(From Samei E. Performance of digital radiographic detectors: factors affecting sharpness and noise. 2003 Syllabus: categorical course in diagnostic radiology physics—advances in digital radiography. Oak Brook, Ill: Radiological Society of North America, 2003; 49-61.)*

as light-directing tubes, much like fiber optics (Figure 5-5). Because of how the cesium iodide crystals are grown, they are considered a structured scintillator. These needles can be evaporated onto the surface of the layer, or they can be grown with a seed layer. This allows greater detection of x-rays (higher detective quantum efficiency DQE than a Gd_2O_2S scintillator), and because there is almost no light spread, the spatial resolution is higher (Figure 5-6). These needles absorb the x-ray photons and convert their energy into light, channeling it to the amorphous silicon photodiode array. In the past, CsI detectors could not be practically used in a portable-type detector. The crystalline structure was too delicate to be used outside of a protected environment of a fixed detector array. However, today, because of the advances in materials and crystalline formation on the array, both CsI and Gd_2O_2S are being used in portable detectors.

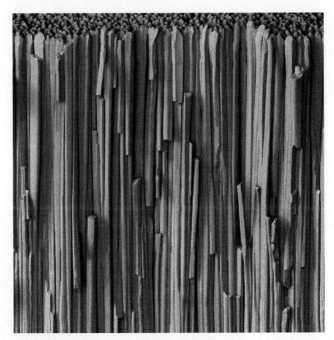

FIGURE 5-5 Cesium iodide crystal structure used in CsI detectors. *(Photo courtesy Dr. Reiner F. Schulz, Seimens Medical Solutions, Vacuum Technology Division.)*

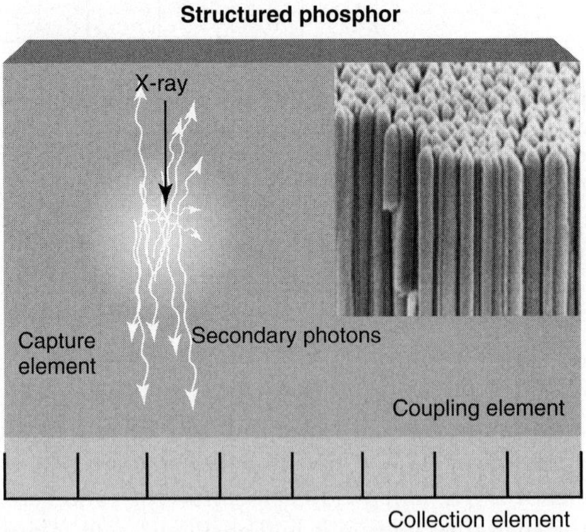

FIGURE 5-6 Cesium Iodide Scintillator Showing Light Spread Potential. *(From Samei E. Performance of digital radiographic detectors: factors affecting sharpness and noise. 2003 Syllabus: categorical course in diagnostic radiology physics—advances in digital radiography. Oak Brook, Ill: Radiological Society of North America, 2003; 49-61.)*

FLAT-PANEL ARRAY DESIGN AND PERFORMANCE

Design

The way an a-Si:H array functions is very complex; however, the design is fairly simple. Each pixel contains a **sensing component** and a **switching component**. There are two types of switching components: a 2-contact switching diode and a 3-contact TFT. The sensing component depends on the type of absorbing material and the vendor's choice of construction. A phosphor/scintillator requires a photodiode or phototransistor to detect the light. If a photoconductor (a-Se) is selected, the sensing element is a capacitor that measures charge. This is also known as a storage capacitor.

To operate, the flat-panel detectors use about 2.5 kilometers or 1.6 miles of electrical bias (a predetermined amount of voltage or current in an electrical circuit), control, and signal output lines laid out on the array surfaces so that each pixel is monitored and refreshed during the control and reading process. Each row of pixels is connected to the same horizontal control line, and each column is connected to the same vertical data line. The readout electronics are attached to the edges of the array, and the entire array and its components are enclosed in a protective housing.

When the exposure is made, the sensing/storage component within the pixel contains the image information. The information is then read out line by line via the changing of the control line voltage so each pixel is connected to its corresponding data line at the bottom of the column (Figure 5-7). Figure 5-7A illustrates the detector in its initialized state, prepared and waiting for exposure. In Figure 5-7B, the detector has been exposed and is awaiting reading of the array. Figure 5-7C demonstrates the readout or release of signal of row one. Notice that a voltage is applied across the control or switch line corresponding to row one. In the final image of Figure 5-7, row one has returned to an initialized state (the process of returning to this state varies per vendor and is beyond the scope of this textbook) after release of its signal and the readout process continues to row two. Once the signal has been released, the energy is then transferred to the electronics that are attached to the edges of the array.

Performance

There are two ways to measure detector performance: (1) numerical measurement of spatial resolution and DQE, and (2) observation of low-contrast objects in a contrast detail phantom. The actual procedures to measure detector performance are beyond the scope of this book; however, current performance measurement of signal-to-noise ratio and DQE support that flat-panel a-Si:H detectors perform better than other digital imaging systems.

FLAT-PANEL ARTIFACTS

Dead Pixels

There is a possibility in any imaging system of losing or misrepresenting image information because of defects in the operation components of the device. Although

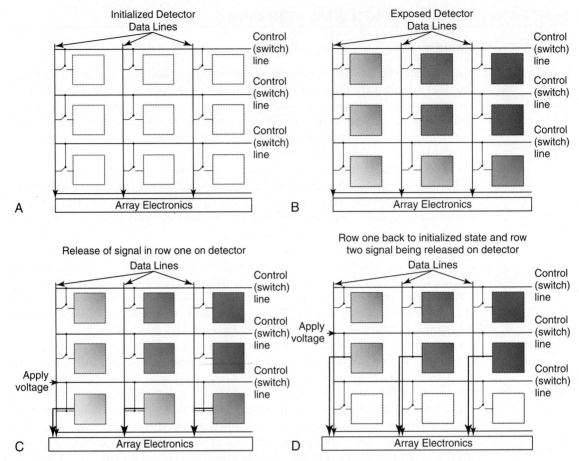

FIGURE 5-7 Detector Readout.

not very common, **image artifacts** can be caused by malfunctions in the detector. Because manufacture of the pixels is so complex, it is inevitable that the array structure will suffer some damage. Dust, scratches, static discharge, chemical corrosion, or interactions between materials can occur, resulting in some defective pixels. These pixels may be malfunctioning or dead, that is, not functioning at all. As the detector ages, the number of dead pixels increases but may not be detected if they are located on the edges of the panel. Manufacturers make efforts to maintain a standard of less than approximately 0.1% to 0.2% defective pixels and build software programs into their systems to identify and isolate dead pixels. The software uses an interpolation method to "fill in" the dead pixels with information using the surrounding pixels as a guide.

Incorrect Gain Calibration

Gain calibration is used to correct flaws in the detector. If an area of the detector has a large amount of dead pixels or if there is an area of the detector that has poor

FIGURE 5-8 Incorrect Gain Calibration Performed. *(Reprinted with permission from the American Journal of Roentgenology.)*

connections between the conversion layer and the a-Si/TFT array, a noticeable artifact can be seen on the screen. To remove the potential of having that artifact interfere with diagnosis, a process known as gain calibration or flat fielding is used. This process will remove these densities on the image by creating a mask of those defects. When a subsequent image is taken, the software will use the mask to remove the unwanted densities and leave only the diagnostic information. Gain calibration should be performed under the same or similar circumstances in which clinical images will be taken. The calibration should be done according to the equipment manufacturer's guidelines. In Figure 5-8, the automatic exposure control AEC cells appear as slightly positive squares in the image. The gain calibration was performed with the detector outside of the Bucky and then a subsequent image was taken with the detector in the Bucky. This could happen if anything is left on the detector during a gain calibration. These faint marks could lead to a misdiagnosis.

Image Lag and Incorrect Offset Correction

Some flat-panel systems have the ability to take images faster than the detector can accommodate. If an image is taken prior to the detector releasing all of the signal from the previous image, a faint image of the previous exposure may be visible. This is known as **image lag**. Image lag is almost a double exposure of sorts. When the detector is unable to get rid of all of the signal from the previous image, lag can occur. Rapid succession of images is only one reason for image lag. Another reason image lag might occur is overexposure or an area with little beam attenuation, such as a technologist's lead marker location. In Figure 5-9, a faint *R* is visible in the proximal thoracic spinous processes. The *R* is left over from the previous image. The following techniques can be used to reduce the possibility of image lag:

- Increase the amount of time between exposures, giving the detector sufficient time to release all of the residual image. Consult the equipment's operator's manual for suggested image intervals.

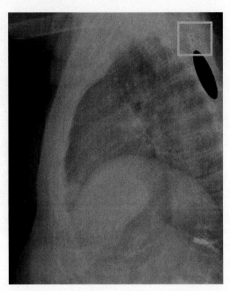

FIGURE 5-9 Example of Image Lag. Notice the faint *R* in the proximal thoracic spinous processes. *(Reprinted with permission from the American Journal of Roentgenology.)*

- Reduce the amount of unattenuated beam by collimating as closely as allowable.
- Set appropriate technical factors for each body part being examined. If multiple examinations are being done, acquire the image requiring the highest technical factors last.

Image lag can also be corrected with the detector's software using the dark noise or offset correction. **Offset correction** determines the amount of signal inherent in the detector. If an offset correction is performed prior to residual signal leaving the pixels, that information will be stored as inherent and could cause a negative image of the residual signal. Always follow the equipment manufacturer's guidelines when performing any detector calibrations. For example, in Figure 5-10 an offset correction was performed after an examination was done with a right side marker in an area of unattenuated radiation. Residual signal remained in that area and a subsequent offset correction was performed. The *R* is now viewed inversely because that signal created a mask during the offset correction. In Figure 5-10 it is clear that the signal is still very strong and this image was taken 10 minutes after the initial exposure.

EMERGING TECHNOLOGY

In conventional projection imaging in the past an imaging technique called tomography was used. Tomograms were acquired by attaching a fulcrum to the Bucky and tubehead. The Bucky and tubehead would move in concert with one another and the tube would arc across the patient. The fulcrum point would determine the area in the body imaged. This same concept is now being used in digital imaging

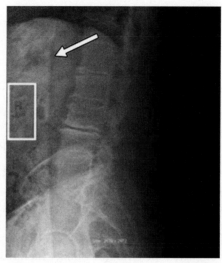

FIGURE 5-10 Image Lag. *(Reprinted with permission from the American Journal of Roentgenology.)*

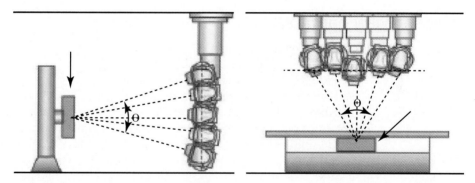

FIGURE 5-11 Detector Lag. *(From Machida H, Yuhara T, Mori T, et al. Optimizing parameters for flat-panel detector digital tomosynthesis.* Radiographics *2010;30:549-562.)*

and it is called tomosynthesis (Figure 5-11). Tomosynthesis was not possible on earlier versions of digital detectors because they were not able to acquire images rapidly in succession. With advances in the selenium detector and amorphous silicon TFT arrays, the detector is now able to acquire images at a rate of 30 frames per second. After the acquisition of the entire set of frames required for the body part being imaged, the frames are sent to a postprocessing workstation for reconstruction. The images are then sent to a viewing station as a stack of images similar to a stack of computed tomography (CT) images. The images can be viewed as single slices or in a cine mode like CT.

Currently most tomosynthesis is being done in breast imaging. It is primarily being used on patients with very dense breast tissue. There have been several studies done looking at the benefit of this type of imaging on the extremities and chest. As the technology becomes more readily available, more applications will be put into use in this imaging modality.

SUMMARY

- There are two types of conversion methods used in TFT flat-panel technology: direct and indirect.
- Direct sensors are TFT arrays of amorphous silicon coated with amorphous selenium (a-Se).
- Direct sensors absorb x-ray photons and immediately convert them to an electrical signal.
- Indirect conversion detectors use a scintillator that converts x-rays into visible light, which is then converted into an electric charge that is collected by a field effect transistor (FET) or silicon TFT.
- Incomplete transfer of the signal generated in the detector or the amount of signal retained by the detector can cause artifacts, especially with short acquisition or rapid succession acquisitions.

CHAPTER REVIEW QUESTIONS

1. A photo conductor:
   a. Produces light when absorbing x-rays.
   b. Produces x-rays when absorbing light.
   c. Absorbs light and produces electric charges.
   d. Absorbs x-rays and produces electrical charges.
2. Which of the following are *not* considered scintillators?
   a. Gd_2O_2S
   b. CsI
   c. a-Se
   d. None of the above
3. Which of the following is used as a photodetector?
   a. Gd_2O_2S
   b. CsI
   c. a-Se
   d. a-Si:H
4. Which of the following are *not* found in an AMFPI?
   a. a-Si TFT with CsI
   b. a-Se with TFT
   c. PSP
   d. Scintillator
5. Which detector(s) converts x-ray energy directly into electrons?
   a. a-Si TFT with CsI
   b. a-Se with TFT
   c. a-Si TFT with Gd_2O_2S
   d. All of the above

6. A Gd_2O_2S scintillator is known as what type of phosphor?
   a. Turbid
   b. Unstructured
   c. Structured
   d. Both A and B
   e. Both A and C

7. Gain calibration will remove inherent detector artifacts from an image.
   a. True
   b. False

8. Offset correction is used to remove inherent signal that remains in a detector.
   a. True
   b. False

9. Which of the following can be done to decrease the chance of having image lag occur in the next image?
   a. Decrease the amount of time between exposures.
   b. Increase the amount of time between exposures.
   c. Leave collimation open.
   . Acquire the image requiring the highest technical factors first.

10. Which type of absorbing material requires a capacitor as the storage element?
    a. a-Se
    b. Photoconductor
    c. Scintillator
    d. Both A and B

CCD/CMOS Image Capture

Polysilicon layer

Silicon dioxide layer

P-type transistors

Silicon substrate

Quantum efficiency

Spectrum sensitivity

Semiconductor

Statistical noise

CHARGE-COUPLED DEVICES (CCDS)

The oldest indirect-conversion digital radiography systems used **charge-coupled devices (CCDs)** to acquire the digital image. These devices are still being used in a variety of image capture applications. In a CCD system, x-ray photons interact with a scintillation material and the signal is transmitted by lenses or fiber optics to the CCD. During the transmission process, the lenses reduce the size of the projected visible light image and transfer the image to one or more small capacitors that convert the light into an electrical charge. This charge is stored in a sequential pattern and released line by line and sent to an **analog-to-digital converter (ADC)** (Figure 6-1).

Structure and Function

A photosensitive receptor and electronics embedded into a substrate material in a silicon chip make up a CCD. Incident light from a scintillator strikes the detector and electron/hole pairs are produced in the silicon. The number of electron/hole pairs is related to the amount of light that is absorbed. The electrons are held by electrostatic forces in the array until the charge is read out to form the image. The chip is made up of a polysilicon layer, a silicon dioxide layer, and a silicon substrate (Figure 6-2). The **polysilicon layer** is coated with a photosensitive material and contains the electronic gates. The **silicon dioxide layer** is an insulator and the **silicon substrate** contains the charge storage area.

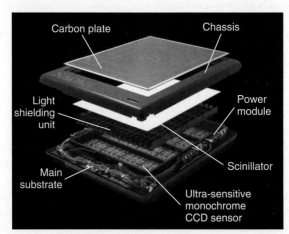

FIGURE 6-1 Multi-CCD Detector Unit. *(Courtesy RF SYSTEM lab/RF Co., Ltd.)*

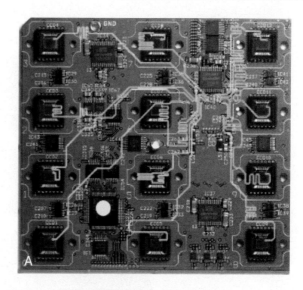

CCD Sense Element (Pixel) Structure

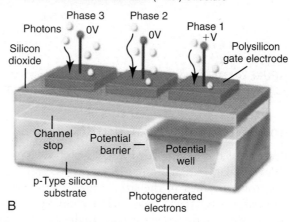

FIGURE 6-2 A, 12-CCD array. **B,** Simplified illustration demonstrating the layers of a CCD chip. (**A** *courtesy RF SYSTEM lab/RF Co., Ltd.* **B** *Courtesy Molecular Expressions (http://microscopy.fsu .edu.)*

Each pixel or **detector element (del)** contains three electrodes that hold the electrons in a electrical potential well. The dels are formed by voltage gates that, at readout, are opened and closed like gates to allow the flow of electrons. To collect the charge on the silicon chips, the voltage sign is changed on the electrodes within each del, moving the electrons by rows down the columns until the readout row is reached. This process is commonly known as the "**bucket brigade scheme**" (Figure 6-3). Once the readout row is reached, the data are sent sequentially to the sense amplifier and are then digitized. The readout process requires that the movement of the electrons is timed, and multiple voltage changes occur; however, the process is very quick. There can be issues with overfill in the dels, which causes excess electrons to spill out of the del into an adjacent del. This is handled by building overflow drains into the array to reduce or prevent this "**blooming**" effect.

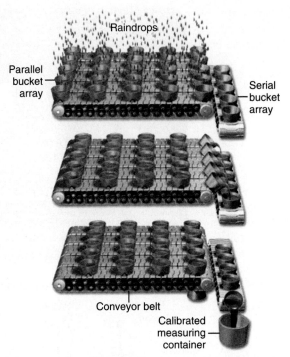

FIGURE 6-3 **The "Bucket Brigade Scheme."** In a process that involves applying varying voltages to each pixel, the pixels are read column by column. *(Courtesy Hamamatsu Photonics.)*

Image-Related Characteristics

Because of the high cost of a CCD chip, it is not practical to manufacture CCD chips any larger than 5 cm × 5 cm. Most chips range from 2 to 4 cm. The image has to be matched to the size of the CCD, which implies that the image must be reduced in size. To do this, CCD technology uses lenses or fiber optics so that the image matches the receptor size. Reducing the image size involves several factors that contribute to the quality of the image and each must be considered. These factors include the scintillator, light collection components, and noise.

The Scintillator. The type of scintillator and the way it is constructed will determine how much of the incident x-ray photons are absorbed, how much light is produced, and the wavelength or color of the light. Remember from Chapter 5 that there are two main types of phosphors: structured and unstructured (turbid). An unstructured phosphor will produce more light spread when stimulated by x-rays, thereby decreasing the efficiency of the detector. Gadolinium oxysulphide (Gd_2O_2S) is considered an unstructured phosphor because of its powderlike grains and cesium iodide (CsI) is considered a structured phosphor because of its needlelike crystals.

CCD systems may use the same scintillator as amorphous silicon technology thin-film transistors (TFTs); CsI is a particularly common scintillator. The CsI needles focus light onto a very narrow area, reducing light spread and allowing the use of thicker scintillators without losing too much spatial resolution.

Lenses and Fiber Optics. Lenses or fiber optics are used to focus light onto the CCD chip. The efficiency of the transportation of light to the chip becomes very important because of the noise created. The more light that is sent to the chip without the creation of noise, the more efficient the system is. The design of the optics is crucial in imaging performance because of the issues that arise with geometric distortion such as light scattering or lens or optics flaws. The ways that physicists and manufacturers determine the efficiency of lenses and fiber optics involve complicated mathematical formulas that are beyond the scope of this text. However, it is important to acknowledge that optics in a CCD are critical contributors to the quality of a digital image and must be considered when evaluating image capture technology.

Detective Quantum Efficiency. The amount of electrons produced relative to the incident light from the scintillator is the **quantum efficiency** of the CCD. The quantum efficiency represents the absolute efficiency of the light collection and the signal created in the chip. This is not detective quantum efficiendy (DQE; ratio of output signal to signal-to-noise ratio), but quantum efficiency does have an effect on DQE.

The CCD device is built to be as efficient as possible. The polysilicon layer must be transparent enough so that light passes through it to reach deeper into the substrate storage area, but not so deep that it cannot be captured in the potential well. Also, the **spectrum sensitivity** of the CCD must match the spectral output of the phosphor. The less sensitive the CCD is to the light spectrum of the scintillator, the less efficient the CCD is.

Noise. There are several types of noise associated with CCD technology; statistical noise, "dark" current noise, and amplification noise are three common types.

Statistical noise is noise created by the lack of light photons from the scintillator. If there are not enough x-ray photons striking the scintillator, or if too few light photons are produced by the scintillator, then too few electrons will be generated and the output signal will be noisy (quantum mottle). **Dark current noise** occurs when the CCD chip operates without radiation stimulation. This happens when the temperature rises and electrons are moved into the bulk silicon or depletion area and are stored until readout occurs later, adding unnecessary information to the image. Some manufacturers add a thermoelectric cooling device that can reduce the temperature as much as 40°F lower than room temperature. Because dark noise can be as much as 10,000 electrons/pixel per second, and a 40° drop can reduce dark noise by a factor of 100, temperature consideration is very important.

Amplification noise is common to digital systems. Even though a CCD is one chip, the process of manufacturing that chip is extremely complicated and the response of each chip will vary across the array. Some pixels may not work at all and although software is used to correct the statistical variation because of inoperable pixels, the more bad pixels, the worse the detector efficiency. Because the manufacturing process is so complex, there are no CCDs without amplification noise; however, the number of defects rises as manufacturing costs decrease. The lower the cost of the CCD, the higher the number of defects.

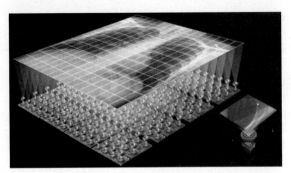

FIGURE 6-4 **Multi-CCD Detector.** *(Courtesy RF SYSTEM lab/RF Co., Ltd.)*

CCD Applications

CCDs are used in several applications in radiology including digital fluoroscopy, stereotactic breast biopsy, digital mammography, and general radiography. In digital fluoroscopy, the CCD is a great replacement for the television (TV) pickup tube in an image intensifier because the CCD size (2 to 5 cm) is closely matched with the output phosphor of an image intensifier (1 inch). The CCD readout is linear and has a greater dynamic range than a TV tube; because oversaturation is almost zero, blooming is greatly reduced, shortening the recovery time from one image to another. CCDs are much more compact than TV tubes and CCDs are not susceptible to electron scanning errors the way that TV tubes are.

For stereotactic breast biopsy applications, a single CCD detector can be used because the typical field size is 50 mm × 50 mm. However, most current systems use a 2.5 cm × 2.5 cm chip that results in some demagnification. Demagnification is the process of reducing the phosphor output image to the size of the active area of the CCD chip. The demagnification uses lenses, optics, and mirrors to accomplish this task. Because of the low dose, noise is not much of a factor. In digital mammography, early applications used CCDs, but these applications are being replaced by flat-panel systems.

In general radiography, CCDs may be tiled in a 16 × 12 array (Figure 6-4) to a single CCD. CsI is common as the scintillation material. Another way CCDs are used is in a whole-body scanner, where 12 CCD cameras are coupled to **gadolinium sulfur dioxide scintillators** with tapered fiber optics. The tube and receptor array are housed in a C-arm type of mount and the body is scanned by a moving fan-beam (slot-scanning device) down the length of the table. The scan can be any length up to 180 cm. The table is actually a stretcher and is largely used for trauma applications and forensic pathology.

CCD Advantages and Disadvantages

CCDs are relatively inexpensive compared to TFT-based flat-panel systems and much more simple. They are modular, making them easy to repair, replace, and upgrade. Advantages and disadvantages depend greatly on the application as noted previously. The strongest advantage of CCDs is their modular design, and the greatest disadvantage relates to demagnification issues and reduced DQE because of the demagnification.

COMPLEMENTARY METAL OXIDE SEMICONDUCTOR (CMOS) SYSTEMS

Developed by NASA, **complementary metal oxide semiconductor (CMOS)** systems use a scintillator that, when struck with x-ray photons, convert the x-rays into light photons and store them in capacitors (Figure 6-5). Each pixel or detector element has its own amplifier, which is switched on and off by circuitry within the pixel, converting the light photons into electrical charges.

Voltage from the amplifier is converted by an ADC. This system is highly efficient and takes up less fill space than CCDs. CMOS is a semiconductor. A **semiconductor** is a solid chemical element or compound that conducts electricity under some conditions but not others, making it a good medium for the control of electrical current. Its ability to conduct current varies depending on the amount of current or voltage it receives or on the intensity of radiation by x-rays. Impurities (also known as

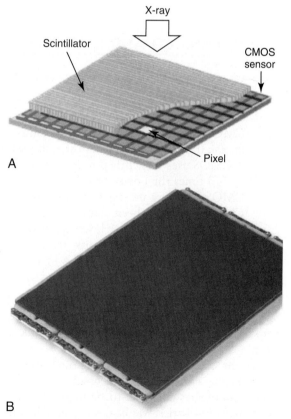

FIGURE 6-5 Simple CMOS Detector. (*A* courtesy RIKEN and JASRI. *B* courtesy Teledyne DALSA.)

dopants) are added to semiconductors because the materials semiconductors are made from do not conduct electricity very well by themselves. Thus they are "doped" with impurities that make them highly conductive.

Typical semiconductor materials are antimony, arsenic, boron, carbon, germanium, selenium, silicon, sulfur, and tellurium. Silicon is the most popular and is the base material of most integrated circuits. Common impurities added to the silicon are gallium arsenide, indium antimonide, and oxides of most metals. When doped, the semiconductor becomes a full-scale conductor or becomes an **N-type transistor** (extra electrons with a negative charge) or positive charge carriers (**P-type transistors**). In most semiconductors of the CMOS kind, both types of transistor are used so that they form a gate that can be controlled electrically. Although CMOS transistors use little to no power when they are not in use, if the direction of the current changes rapidly, the transistors become hot and this slows down the microprocessors.

Like CCD technology, CMOS image sensors convert light into electrons. The electrons are stored in capacitors located within the pixel. During readout, the charge is sent across the chip and read at one corner of the array. This is typically done using several transistors at each pixel that amplify the charge and send it through wires to the array corner. An ADC turns each pixel's value into a digital value.

COMPARISON BETWEEN CCD AND CMOS TECHNOLOGY

There are some noticeable differences between CCD and CMOS sensors.

- CMOS sensors are more susceptible to noise.
- Light sensitivity of a CMOS chip is lower than a CCD. This is because the CMOS pixels are surrounded with transistors and many of the light photons hit the transistors rather than the photodiode.
- A CMOS uses very little power compared to a CCD. CCDs may use as much as 110 times the power that CMOSs use.
- CMOSs are very inexpensive to manufacture compared to CCD sensors.
- CMOS chips have been manufactured for a shorter period of time than CCD sensors and tend to have lower quality, lower resolutions, and lower sensitivity. However, CMOS sensors are quickly improving, and their quality is almost as good as that of CCDs in some applications.
- The pixel fill factor is greater with CCDs than CMOSs.

Despite their differences CCD and CMOS technologies both provide excellent image capture capabilities; also for both, their usefulness depends on the type of application. Each has strengths unique to those applications and neither is superior to the other.

Current CMOS designers are working diligently to increase image quality and CCD designers are seeking to decrease power requirements and pixel sizes. Both of these technologies continue to be improved year after year because of their wide use in many industries. Medical imaging will continue to see growth and new applications from both CCD and CMOS detectors.

SUMMARY

- A charge-coupled device (CCD) acts as a receptor that senses light generated in a scintillator and then sends the light to capacitors in the pixel that converts light to an electrical charge. The charge is released line by line and sent to an analog-to-digital converter (ADC), and the digital signal is sent for processing.
- The type and construction of the scintillator, as well as the lenses of fiber optic components, affect spatial resolution and noise.
- Quantum efficiency of CCD technology is a measure of the efficiency of the light collection and the signal created in the CCD chip.
- The spectrum sensitivity of a CCD has to match the spectral output of the phosphor in order to gain the greatest efficiency.
- Three types of noise—statistical, dark current, and amplification—were discussed. Light photon production, insufficient incident radiation, broken or inoperable pixels, and temperature are significant contributing factors to noise.
- CCD technology has applications in digital fluoroscopy, stereotactic breast biopsy, digital mammography, and general radiography. CCDs are relatively inexpensive and simple.
- Complementary metal oxide semiconductor (CMOS) systems use scintillators that, when struck with x-ray photons, convert the x-rays into light photons and store them in capacitors. Each pixel's amplifier is switched on and off, converting light photons into electrical charges. Charges are fed to an ADC and are released at readout.
- Highly efficient and small, a CMOS is a semiconductor that consists of a material (such as antimony, boron, silicon, etc.) doped with an impurity such as gallium arsenide or a metal oxide. The impurity makes the semiconductor a full electrical conductor or the excess electrons become negative or positive (N-type or P-type) transistors. These transistors can be controlled electrically, forming gates to change charge direction.

CHAPTER REVIEW QUESTIONS

1. A charge-coupled device (CCD) does all of the following *except*:
   a. Reduce the size of the projected light image
   b. Transfer the image to a capacitor
   c. Convert light into x-ray photons
   d. Act as receptors via lenses or fiber optics
2. The number of electron/hole pairs is related to the amount of:
   a. Light absorbed
   b. Electric charge
   c. Incident x-rays
   d. Reflected light
3. The layer in a CCD chip that contains the electron gates is the:
   a. Silicon dioxide layer
   b. Polysilicon layer
   c. Silicon substrate
   d. All of the above

4. The insulating layer in a CCD chip is the:
   a. Polygonal layer
   b. Silicon substrate
   c. Silicon dioxide layer
   d. Monosilicon layer
5. A system that used scintillators that convert x-rays to light, light to electric charge, and store the charge in capacitors is known as a:
   a. CCD
   b. ADC
   c. Image intensifier
   d. CMOS
6. A solid chemical element or compound doped with impurities that make it highly conductive is known as a:
   a. Dopant
   b. Semiconductor
   c. Transistor
   d. Capacitor
7. Most CMOS detectors use both N-type and P-type transistors to form the electrically controlled gate.
   a. True
   b. False
8. Which of the two technologies, CCDs or CMOS, is more susceptible to noise, has a lower light sensitivity, uses very little power, and is inexpensive to manufacture?
   a. CCD
   b. CMOS

PART IV

Picture Archiving and Communication Systems (PACS)

Basic Computer Principles

OBJECTIVES

On completion of this chapter, you should be able to:
- Describe the major components of a computer.
- Define binary code, bit, and byte, and discuss how they relate to one another.
- List and define the hardware components discussed in this chapter.
- List the three most common types of monitors.
- Explain the measurements used to classify monitors.
- Compare and contrast an operating system and application software.
- Discuss the uses of computers in a radiology department.

OUTLINE

How Does the Computer Work?
Hardware Components
  The Case
  The Motherboard
  Sound Card
  Network Card
  Hard Drive
  CD/DVD Drive
  Peripherals
Monitors
  CRT
  LCD
  Monitor Advantages and Disadvantages
Operating Systems
Computers in the Radiology Department
Summary

KEY TERMS

Aspect ratio	Dot pitch
Binary code	Hard drive
Basic input/output system (BIOS)	Memory
Bit	Motherboard
Bus	Operating system (OS)
Byte	Port
Central processing unit (CPU)	Power supply
Complementary metal oxide	Refresh rate
semiconductor (CMOS)	Resolution
Computer	Viewable area

A **computer** is a programmable electronic device that can store, retrieve, and process data. This chapter provides an overview of how a computer works, the basic hardware components of a computer system, the differences between each type of system, and the different types of monitors. An understanding of these basic topics will provide a foundation for the discussion in the following chapters of picture archiving and communication (PAC) and digital radiographic systems.

HOW DOES THE COMPUTER WORK?

In its basic form, a computer consists of input, output, and processing devices (Figure 7-1). Input devices are keyboards, mice, microphones, barcode readers, touch screens, and image scanners, and any of these can be found in a modern radiology department. Common output devices are monitors, printers, and speakers. The computer also has various communication devices that it uses to share information. The processing of information is done in the central processing unit, which will be detailed later in the chapter.

The computer takes data from the user and processes it using a machine language of 1s and 0s, known as **binary code**. The computer processing is performed by a

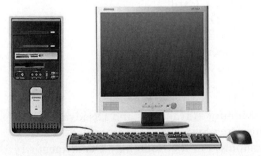

FIGURE 7-1 A Basic Personal Computer Consisting of a CPU, Keyboard, Mouse, and LCD Monitor.

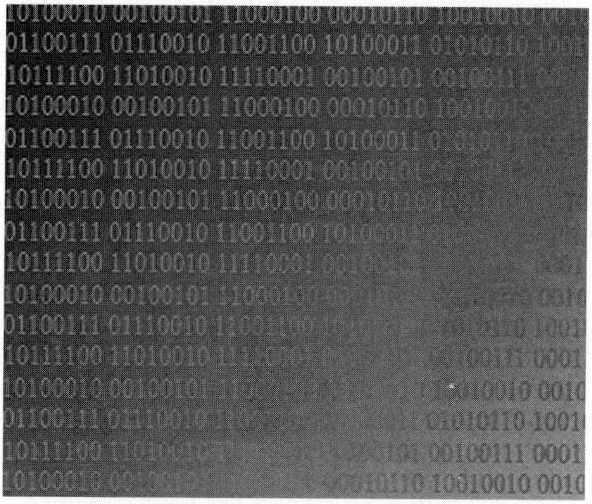

FIGURE 7-2 Binary Code Consists of 1s and 0s.

series of transistors, which are switches that are either on or off (Figure 7-2). If the transistor circuit is closed and current passes through, it is assigned a value of 1. If no current passes because the circuit is open, it is assigned a value of 0. A computer's transistors can be switched on and off millions of times in a second. Each 1 and each 0 represents a bit. A **bit** is a single unit of data. A **byte** is made up of eight bits and is the amount of memory needed to store one alphanumeric character (Figure 7-3). Because one character takes up a byte of memory, memory is generally talked about in kilobytes, megabytes, gigabytes, and even terabytes.

HARDWARE COMPONENTS

The Case

The computer encasement is made from a heavy metal and has two major functions:

1. To hold all of the components in a relatively cool, clean, and safe environment
2. To shield the outside environment from the radio frequencies being emitted by the electronic components of the computer

The case comes in two major configurations: the desktop model and the tower (Figure 7-4). The desktop model is generally positioned in a horizontal encasement, whereas a tower model is in a vertical encasement. As the name implies, most desktop models are placed on the desk underneath the monitor. The tower model is generally placed underneath the desk within arm's reach of the operator. The biggest disadvantages of the desktop model are (1) the space it takes up on the desk and (2) having less room for expansion and upgrades because of the smaller encasement. The tower model consistently provides adequate room for expansion of components, and it is easily placed out of the way and off the work surface.

Letter	Binary code
A	01000001
B	01000010
C	01000011
D	01000100
E	01000101
F	01000110
G	01000111
H	01001000
I	01001001
J	01001010
K	01001011
L	01001100
M	01001101
N	01001110
O	01001111
P	01010000
Q	01010001
R	01010010
S	01010011
T	01010100
U	01010101
V	01010110
W	01010111
X	01011000
Y	01011001
Z	01011010

Letter	Binary code
a	01100001
b	01100010
c	01100011
d	01100100
e	01100101
f	01100110
g	01100111
h	01101000
i	01101001
j	01101010
k	01101011
l	01101100
m	01101101
n	01101110
o	01101111
p	01110000
q	01110001
r	01110010
s	01110011
t	01110100
u	01110101
v	01110110
w	01110111
x	01111000
y	01111001
z	01111010

FIGURE 7-3 **Binary Representation of the Alphabet.**

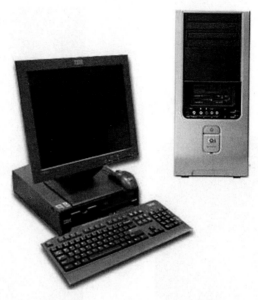

FIGURE 7-4 The desktop model is pictured on the left, and the tower is pictured on the right.

The Motherboard

The **motherboard** (Figure 7-5) is the largest circuitry board inside the computer, and it contains many important small components to make the computer function properly. This chapter covers only a few of the motherboard's components in detail: the CPU, basic input/output system (BIOS), bus, memory, ports, and complementary metal oxide semiconductor (CMOS).

The CPU. Many people refer to the personal computer's (PC) encasement as the CPU. This is incorrect. The **central processing unit (CPU)**, or microprocessor, is a small chip found on the motherboard (Figure 7-6). The microprocessor is the brain of the computer. It consists of a series of transistors that are arranged to manipulate data received from the software.

Microprocessors come in many different sizes and speeds and are manufactured by two major companies, Intel and Advanced Micro Devices (AMD). The CPU's basic tasks are to read data from storage, manipulate the data, and then move the data back to storage or send it to external devices, such as monitors or printers.

The microprocessor is named after its manufacturer and the speed at which it manipulates data. The first microprocessor to be placed in a computer was made in 1979 by Intel and was called the 8088.

It had a clock speed of a mere 4.77 MHz. The more modern Pentium 4 microprocessor has speeds upward of 3.2 to 3.8 GHz. To put these speeds in perspective, the 8088 needed about 12 cycles to complete one basic instruction, and the modern Pentium processor can complete one instruction per cycle.

The BIOS. The **basic input/output system (BIOS)** contains a simple set of instructions for the computer. The microprocessor uses the BIOS during the boot-up

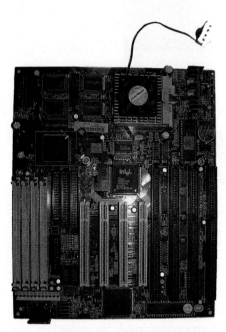

FIGURE 7-5 Motherboard.

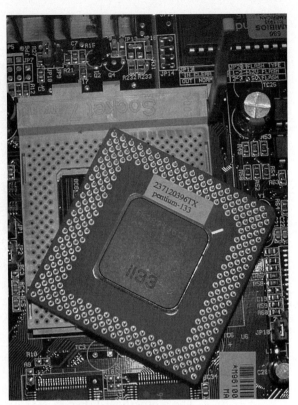

FIGURE 7-6 Central Processing Unit.

process of the computer to help bring the computer to life. The BIOS also runs the start-up diagnostics on the system to make sure all of the peripherals are functioning properly. After the computer has booted up, the BIOS oversees the basic functions of receiving and interpreting signals from the keyboard and interchanging information with various ports. The BIOS is the intermediary between the operating system and the hardware.

The Bus. The **bus** is a series of connections, controllers, and chips that creates the information highway of the computer. There are several buses throughout the computer that connect the microprocessor, the system memory, and various peripherals. Most modern PCs have what is called a peripheral component interconnect (PCI) bus on the motherboard to serve as the connection of information to the various adapters. Other buses found within the computer are for the small computer system interface (SCSI) connections, the accelerated graphics port (AGP) for video adapters, and the universal serial bus (USB) for a variety of devices. Simply put, the bus provides the connections for the information to flow within the computer.

Memory. The **memory** in the computer is used to store information currently being processed within the CPU (Figure 7-7). This memory is also known as random access memory (RAM). The RAM is short-term storage for open programs. The microprocessor has a small amount of memory within itself but not enough to tackle the large amounts of data being generated by high-level programs. The RAM will

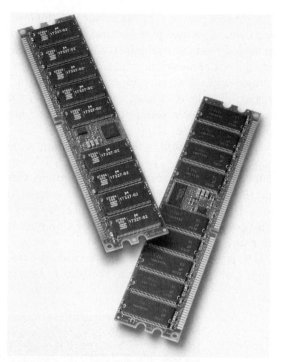

FIGURE 7-7 Memory Chip. *(Courtesy Sun Corporation.)*

take the data from the CPU so that the CPU can handle the processing needs of the programs that are running. The RAM is only temporary; once the computer has been turned off, the RAM is wiped clean. With today's complex programs and graphics, computers require more memory to function at an acceptable level. There are many different types of RAM available: DRAM, EDO RAM, VRAM, SRAM, SDRAM, SIMM, DIMM, and ECO. Most modern PCs have an SDRAM-DDR, specifically DDR3 SDRAM (double data rate type three synchronous dynamic random access memory). Memory is measured in bytes and can be found in configurations such as 4 gigabytes (GB), 8 GB, 12 GB, and so on. In 1975 the Altair 8800 came with 0.25 kilobytes (KB) of memory at a cost of $103; at that price, 1 gigabyte would cost approximately $432 million. With more modern pricing, one can purchase 4 GB of DDR3 for approximately $25, which equates to $6.25 per gigabyte. These figures are given for perspective purposes and become quickly outdated, so please research current memory capacities and prices for up-to-date information.

Ports. The computer's **ports** are a collection of connectors sticking out of the back of the PC that link adapter cards, drives, printers, scanners, keyboards, mice, and other peripherals that may be used. There are many different types of ports, such as parallel, serial, USB, integrated drive electronics (IDE), and small computer system interface (SCSI). We discuss each of these types and how they may be used within a system.

A parallel port is a 25-pin connector (Figure 7-8). The parallel port was synonymous with a printer port because it was most often used for that purpose prior to the widespread use of the USB connection. A parallel port could send 8 bits of data through the connection, whereas a serial port could send only 1 bit of data down a single wire. A serial port can be universally used for many of the components plugged into the computer, such as a mouse, which does not require the speed of a parallel port. Most serial ports are of the 9-pin variety, but some can have up to 25-pin connectors.

A USB connection is the most common wired connection used between devices today (Figure 7-9). The advantage of a USB port is that multiple devices may be connected into one port. In older computers there were only ports for the keyboard and the mouse, one parallel port for a printer, and one serial port for a modem. By using USB ports the user can connect up to 127 devices to one single USB port. Most computers have more than one USB port available, so the possible connections are many.

IDE ports can be found on the motherboard and connect the hard drive, floppy drive, and CD-ROM drive to the board. A series of ribbon cables runs throughout

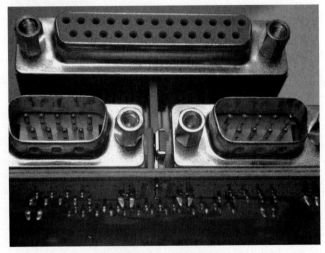

FIGURE 7-8 Parallel Port.

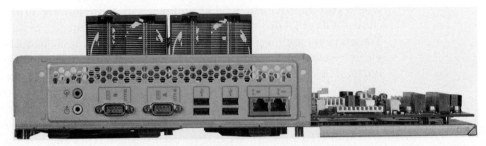

FIGURE 7-9 USB Port. *(Courtesy Sun Corporation.)*

the computer to connect the IDE devices to the IDE port on the motherboard. The fifth type of port is the SCSI port. It is the fastest and most versatile way for a PC to communicate with its peripherals. A single SCSI controller can manage up to seven devices through a daisy chain connection. The most common SCSI devices are hard drives, CD-ROM drives, scanners, and printers.

CMOS. The **complementary metal oxide semiconductor (CMOS)** is a special type of memory chip that uses a small rechargeable or lithium battery to retain information about the PC's hardware while the computer is turned off. The CMOS is also the location of the system clock that keeps track of the date and time. The system clock uses a vibrating quartz crystal to set the speed for the CPU. A single tick of the clock represents the time it takes to turn a transistor on and off. Because modern CPUs are measured in gigahertz, a PC with a 3-GHz CPU has a system clock that ticks 3 billion times per second. Also at bootup, the CMOS chip will detect any changes in the system since the last basic system configuration and will prompt the system to install any new hardware.

Sound Card

The sound card contains all of the circuitry for recording and reproducing sound on the PC. It may be in the form of an expansion card, or it may be built into several chips found on the motherboard. Ports are located externally to connect amplified speakers, headphones, microphone, and a compact disk (CD) player input into the computer. The sound card interprets many file types such as waveform audio (WAV) files, moving picture experts group audio layer 3 (MP3) files, and musical instrument digital interface (MIDI) files.

Network Card

The network interface card (NIC) can come either as an expansion card (Figure 7-10) plugged into a slot or as part of the PC motherboard circuitry. The network card will have an RJ-45 adapter jack (Figure 7-11) at the rear of the PC for the acceptance of a twisted-pair wire with RJ-45 connector (Figure 7-12). This network

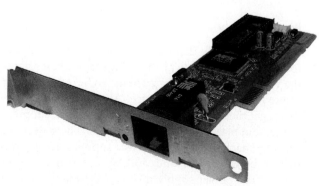

FIGURE 7-10 Network Interface Card (NIC).

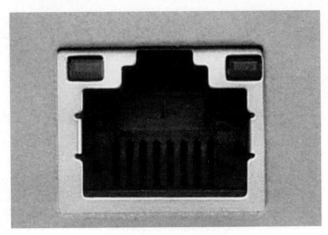

FIGURE 7-11 RJ-45 Jack.

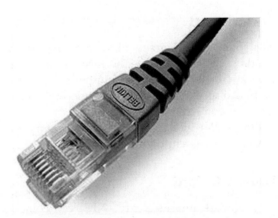

FIGURE 7-12 RJ-45 Connector.

card will enable the PC to connect to other PCs that are on the same network. Detailed information about networks is discussed in the next chapter.

Power Supply

The **power supply** (Figure 7-13) delivers all electricity to the PC and contains a fan to help keep the inside of the computer cool. It contains a transformer that converts the wall outlet alternating current (AC) to direct current (DC) in the voltages appropriate for each powered device. All components, from the motherboard to the hard drive, get their power directly from the main supply through different colored wires that end in plastic shielded connectors. The power supplies deliver ±12 V, ±5 V, and in some machines +3.3 V. Power supplies are rated in watts. Most power supplies deliver between 150 and 300 W, but some computers require a 400-W power supply. The power supply is designed to take the brunt of the force if the computer ever receives a power surge. In such a case, the power supply is easily replaced.

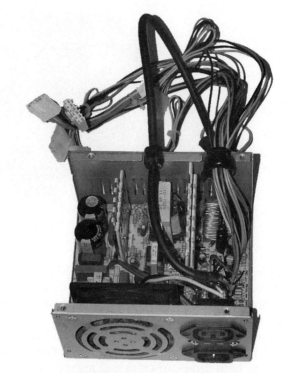

FIGURE 7-13 Power Supply.

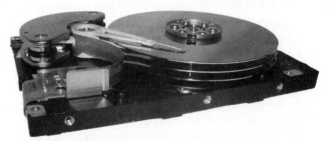

FIGURE 7-14 Looking Inside the Hard Drive.

Hard Drive

The **hard drive** is the main repository for programs and documents on a PC. The hard drive is made up of many hard, thin magnetic platters that are stacked one on top of the other with only enough space for a read-write head to glide over the surface of the disks (Figure 7-14). The disks are spun at a fast speed by a small motor, and the read/write head glides to the area that houses the particular information needed and reads or writes as asked.

The early disks had a storage capacity of 10 MB and could be accessed in approximately 80 ms. In 1980 a 26-MG drive was priced at $5,000. The more

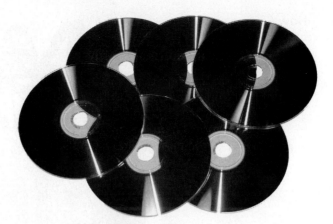

FIGURE 7-15 Compact Disks.

modern disks can hold upward of 3 terabytes (TB) with an access speed of 4 ms at a price of $160. In 1980, this 3 TB of storage would have cost approximately $19.7 million. As storage capacity has skyrocketed, the price per gigabyte of storage has drastically decreased. The drives may be faster than ever, but they are still the slowest part of the PC because they are both mechanical and electrical. These figures were given for perspective purposes and become quickly outdated, so please research current hard drive capacities and prices.

CD/DVD Drive

A compact disk (CD) is a thin injection-molded polycarbonate plastic disk (Figure 7-15). The disk is impressed from a mold to form microscopic bumps that indicate either a 1 or a 0 to the computer. Over the bumps is a reflective layer of aluminum, and over that is a clear protective coat of acrylic. A CD can hold up to 74 minutes of music or approximately 780 MB of data.

A digital versatile disk (DVD) holds up to seven times more than the CD, which equates to about 9.4 (single-sided) to 17 GB (double-sided) of data. A DVD has multiple layers of polycarbonate plastic. Aluminum is used behind the inner layers, and gold is used behind the outer layers. The gold is semireflective so that it allows the laser to penetrate through to the inner layers of plastic.

There are three main types of CD/DVD drives available in today's market: the ROM (read-only memory), the R (write once–read many), and the RW (read and write many times). CD-ROM drives were placed into early computers. Few computers today can be bought with a simple ROM drive installed. Most modern computers have either a CD-RW or a CD/DVD-RW. With an R or RW drive, information that needs to be saved, transported, or archived can be "burned" (information written on a disk). The information is burned onto the disk, starting in the center and spiraling out to the edge of the disk. The laser burns a tiny depression (pit) into the disk to represent the data being saved. A burned disk will be a series of pits and lands, or areas that were not burned by the laser. Two-sided DVDs can be burned on both sides to double the capacity of the disk.

How CD/DVD Drives Work. A CD/DVD drive is found on the front of the encasement of a computer. The drive consists of a disk tray, a motor, a read head, and possibly a write head. The drive has a small door that opens horizontally, and a tray appears for the disk to be placed. After the door closes, a motor constantly varies the speed of the disk so that the portion above the read head spins at a constant speed no matter its location over the disk. The laser beam of the read head penetrates the disk and strikes the reflective layer. If the laser strikes a land area, the light reflects back; if the laser strikes a pit, the light is scattered. The light reflected back is read by a light-sensing diode that translates the impulses into 1s and 0s for the computer to generate into recognizable data.

Peripherals

Keyboard. There are two basic types of keyboards: soft and click. If there is an audible sound when the keys are depressed, it is a click keyboard. The first keyboards made by IBM were click keyboards. Most modern keyboards connect using an IBM programming system 2 (PS/2) connection and connect into the back of the box. Some keyboards use the USB connection because of its versatility and ease of use. With the advent of wireless connections, keyboard makers use either infrared or radio frequency (RF) signals.

When the keys are depressed on the keyboard, a signal is sent through the switch to the motherboard, where it is interpreted in the keyboard microprocessor. Because of all the switches underneath the keys, keyboards should be kept clean, and food and drink should never be consumed near the keyboard.

Mouse. A mouse is a device with two or sometimes three buttons that allow the user to move the computer's cursor to activate and perform functions within the computer's software.

There are five types of mouse connections (all are serial-type connections):

- Serial mouse: uses a standard serial connection
- Bus mouse: uses a dedicated controller card that is connected to the motherboard
- PS/2 mouse: a special connection for mice that does not use the standard serial port
- USB mouse: attaches to a USB port
- Infrared mouse: uses the computer's infrared port (wireless)

There are three types of mice commonly used:

- Mechanical: This mouse uses a hard rubber ball inside an opening on the bottom that is surrounded by sensing devices. The ball moves around based on the movement of the user's hand over the mouse and triggers the sensors within the mouse to move the cursor on the screen.
- Optical: This mouse has a high-intensity diode that bounces light off surfaces and back to a receiver inside the mouse. As with the mechanical mouse, the cursor is made to move by the movements of the mouse over a hard surface and by the light that is reflected back to the sensors within the mouse.

- Optomechanical: This mouse is a hybrid of mechanical and optical mouse. It uses a rubber ball that interacts with rollers that trigger the optical sensors within the mouse. Light is reflected back to the sensors based on the movement of the rollers.

Scanners. Scanners are devices that capture drawings or written paper documents and convert them into a digital image or document that can be edited. Special image scanners in radiology departments are used to convert an analog (film) image into a digital image. The purpose is to provide a way to compare a hard-copy image with a digital image on a PAC system (PACS; see Chapter 10).

Speakers. Speakers receive sound data from a sound card that is either built into the motherboard or is an expansion card. The sound data are converted from an electrical signal to a series of vibrations in the speaker to create sound. Speakers have become an integral part of the modern PC because they give audible signals from the software to alert us to various tasks.

Microphones. Microphones are used to record voice or to use voice dictation software. Voice dictation software is becoming more common in radiology departments. The technology has progressed to a point that most people's voices can be recognized by the system's software.

MONITORS

There are two major types of monitors: the cathode ray tube (CRT) and the liquid crystal display (LCD). A third type just on the horizon is the organic light-emitting diode (OLED). To understand how these monitors work, we must first look at several basic terms and measurements related to onscreen viewing.

A basic picture element on a display is known as a pixel. A pixel is an individual controllable set of dot triads. A dot triad is a grouping of one red dot, one green dot, and one blue dot. The number of pixels on a display is known as its **resolution**. The more pixels in an image, the higher the resolution of the image and the more information can be displayed. Resolution can also be defined as the process or capability of distinguishing between individual parts of an image that are adjacent. Pixels are arranged in a matrix, a rectangular or square table of numbers that represents the pixel intensity to be displayed on the monitor. Common screen resolutions are 1024×768, 1280×1024, 2048×1536 (3 megapixels [mp]), 2048×2560 (5 mp), 2048×3280 (6 mp), and 2560×4096 (10 mp). The last four matrices are common in image viewing applications with the 5-, 6-, and 10-mp monitors truly only needed in digital projection radiography and mammography.

A third measurement is dot pitch. **Dot pitch** is the measurement of how close the dots are located to one another within a pixel; the smaller the dot pitch of a display, the finer the resolution. Dot pitch may be expressed as aperture grille pitch, pixel pitch, or slot pitch, depending on the monitor maker.

Another measurement is the refresh rate for CRT and response rate for LCD. The **refresh rate** is the measure of how fast the monitor rewrites the screen or the number of times that the image is redrawn on the display each second. The refresh rate helps to control the flicker seen by the user; the higher the refresh rate, the less flicker. Response rate refers to the amount of time that it takes the crystal to go from an off state to on and vice versa. A slower response time will cause blurring during the viewing of dynamic images or moving images.

Another set of display terms is aspect ratio and viewable area. The **aspect ratio** is the ratio of the width of the monitor to the height of the monitor. Most CRT monitors have an aspect ratio of 4:3; LCD monitors have a ratio of 16:9. The **viewable area** is measured diagonally from one corner of the display to the opposite corner.

CRT

CRT monitors were used in the first generation of PCs, and this type of monitor continues to be popular (Figure 7-16). The CRT consists of a cathode and anode within a vacuum tube. The CRT works much like an x-ray tube, in that the cathode boils off a cloud of electrons and then a potential difference is placed on the tube. A stream of electrons is sent across to the monitor's anode, which is a sheet of glass coated with a phosphor layer. The electrons strike the phosphor on the glass, causing the glass to emit a color that is determined by the intensity of the interaction and area with which the electrons interacted.

The electrons interact with either a red, green, or blue dot to form the color and image that is being sent from the video card signal. The electron beam starts in the upper left corner and scans across the glass from side to side and top to bottom, and once it reaches the bottom, it starts again at the top left. On average, most monitors have 350 lines to be scanned. Earlier we discussed the refresh rate being 60 to 75 Hz. This equates to 350 lines being scanned 60 to 75 times per second.

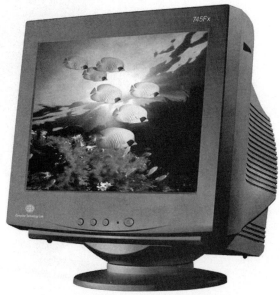

FIGURE 7-16 Cathode Ray Tube (CRT) Monitor.

LCD

An LCD monitor produces images by shining or reflecting light through a layer of liquid crystal and a series of color filters (Figure 7-17). An LCD has two pieces of polarized glass with a liquid crystal material between the two. Light is allowed through the first layer of glass, and when a current is applied to the liquid crystal, it aligns and allows light in varying intensities through to the next layer of glass through color filters to form the colors and images seen on the display. These monitors are particularly effective in brightly lit rooms. One drawback, however, is that LCD monitors are best viewed straight from the monitor surface because the image fades as the viewing angle moves away. Research is ongoing to minimize viewing issues.

Monitor Advantages and Disadvantages

Most consumers want a monitor that can provide the highest resolution for the best price. Table 7-1 outlines the advantages and disadvantages of the two major types of monitors. Historically, most radiology departments used the CRT because of its superior resolution, but LCDs have now taken over health care because they are slimmer and lighter. The LCD monitor has improved many of its early shortcomings to overtake the CRT in medical imaging.

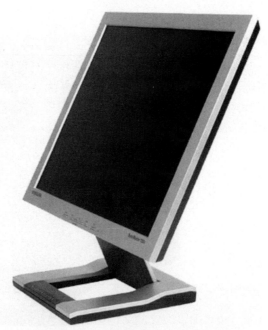

FIGURE 7-17 Liquid Crystal Display (LCD).

TABLE 7-1	Advantages and Disadvantages of CRT and LCD Monitors	
Monitor Type	**Advantages**	**Disadvantages**
CRT		
	Less expensive	Bulky
	Better color representation	The larger the viewing area, the deeper and
	More responsive than LCD	heavier the unit
	Can provide multiple resolutions	Not easily adjusted for viewing at different heights
	More rugged and can sustain rough	and angles
	handling	
LCD		
	Takes up less space than a CRT	Costs more than CRT
	Consumes less power than CRT	Less of a viewing angle
	Produces less heat than CRT	Not as bright as CRT
	Surface produces little or no glare	Each display is capable of working with only one
	Requires a smaller frame around display	physical resolution

CRT, Cathode ray tube; *LCD*, liquid crystal display.

OPERATING SYSTEMS

An **operating system (OS)** is the software that controls the computer hardware and acts as a bridge between applications and the hardware. There are three major OSs in use today: Windows by Microsoft, the Macintosh OS, and UNIX/Linux. PCs generally run a Windows version of an OS, such as Windows 95, 98, 2000, ME, XP, or NT.

There are four types of OSs:

- Real-time OS: used to control specific machinery, scientific instruments, and industrial systems, such as digital x-ray consoles found on modern x-ray equipment.
- Single-user, single-task: designed so that a computer can effectively do one task for one person at a time, such as a Palm OS for the handheld personal organizer.
- Single-user, multitask: designed for one user to perform multiple functions at the same time, such as the OS on a PC.
- Multiuser: designed to handle multiple users and multiple tasks at the same time, such as UNIX running on a large server or as a mainframe computer supporting an entire company.

The computer must have an OS for it to be able to fully function as it was intended. The OS takes over just after the computer wakes up and allows the computer to begin doing tasks. All other software runs using the OS. The various programs that are used on the computer are specifically designed to run on the OS that is loaded on the computer. Early OSs, such as Microsoft–Disk Operating System (MS-DOS), were command based and very difficult to use. The user needed to know word commands to type in to get the computer to do simple tasks, such as saving a file. Today most computers use what is called graphical user interface (GUI) to perform various computer functions. A GUI (goo-ee) is a picture/icon-based program, where the mouse is used to point and click on the function that needs to be performed. The GUI also has easy to use drop-down word menus that can be selected to perform various functions.

As mentioned earlier, IBM-type PCs have traditionally used a Windows-based OS. Large workstations that are used to complete multiple tasks may use Windows NT, or they may use UNIX or Linux for the OS. UNIX is a robust OS. It was first developed by Bell Laboratories and was given out free to universities. It is primarily used by industry for larger server applications. Some PACS vendors began their software on UNIX-based systems but have since migrated to the Windows platform because of cost, ease of use, and customer demand. Linux was derived from UNIX by a Finnish computer science student and is widely used by computer aficionados. Linux is what is known as open-source software; programmers can make changes in the code as long as the changes are shared with others.

All digital medical imaging devices have some sort of OS running behind the user interface. Depending on the vendor, it may be one of the three discussed here or it may be a proprietary (written and known only by the vendor) system developed specifically for a particular device. PACS are no exception. Most modern PACSs use a Windows-based platform, but some may still use UNIX on their large servers because of its exceptional multitasking capabilities.

COMPUTERS IN THE RADIOLOGY DEPARTMENT

Computers are used throughout radiology departments, from the front desk to the file room and from the technologist's work area to the radiologist's reading room. Many computer applications are used throughout the day by the various staff within the department to improve the care that is given to the patient. In most areas, a simple computer can do the job, but in some more complex applications, a specialty workstation is needed to handle the complicated tasks. Most radiology imaging equipment manufactured today has a computer built into the machine itself, or it has a separate computer that is attached for various applications.

Computer hardware and software are chosen to match the applications used by the staff. Comfort, cost, quality, and purpose are four areas that are addressed when choosing the appropriate equipment and accessories. For example, a radiologist would require a monitor with high brightness, high resolution, and a large screen to view digital images for diagnosis, whereas a file room clerk would need only a basic monitor.

At the time of this edition, the iPhone and iPad, Android phones, and tablet PCs are seeing an emergence into health care. Smartphone and personal digital assistant applications can be used to view digital imaging and communications in medicine (DICOM) images, and there are many research studies being performed to better apply this mobile technology. In February 2011 the Food and Drug Administration cleared the first application for diagnosis of computer tomography (CT), magnetic resonance imaging (MRI), and nuclear medicine images on a mobile device. This software application was developed by MIM Software Inc. for Apple's iPhone and iPad products. The application is intended for radiologists and other health care practitioners to use when a full diagnostic workstation is unavailable. Many more applications are anticipated in the future as this technology continues to improve in security and screen resolution.

SUMMARY

- A computer is a programmable electronic device that can store, retrieve, and process data.
- A bit is a single unit of data. There are 8 bits in a byte.
- A computer consists of input, output, and processing devices.
- Input = keyboard, mouse, scanner, barcode reader, and microphone.
- Output = monitor, printer, and speakers.
- Processing = motherboard, microprocessor, basic input/output system (BIOS), bus, memory, ports, and complementary metal oxide semiconductor (CMOS).
- Modern computers contain many types of drives: hard drives, CD-ROM, CD-R, CD-RW, DVD-R, DVD-RW, and floppy. These drives perform specific tasks and functions for the computer.
- Various expansion cards are used within modern PCs: sound cards, network cards, and other peripheral cards.
- Keyboards and mice are the most common input devices. There are various types of each.
- Monitors are measured by several factors: resolution, dot pitch, refresh rate, response rate, aspect ratio, and viewable area.
- There are three types of monitors: CRT, LCD, and OLED.
- An OS is the software that controls the computer hardware and acts as a bridge between applications and hardware.
- Computers are found throughout the radiology department, and each kind has been chosen to fulfill a specific purpose.

CHAPTER REVIEW QUESTIONS

1. A generic term that is used to describe a programmable electronic device that can store, retrieve, and process data is a_____.
   a. Network
   b. Thin-client
   c. Protocol
   d. Computer
2. How many bits are in a single byte?
   a. 0
   b. 1
   c. 8
   d. 16

3. What keeps the radio frequencies generated within the computer electronics from interfering with outside devices?
   a. The case
   b. The motherboard
   c. The CPU
   d. The bus
4. What is the largest circuitry board inside the computer?
   a. CPU
   b. Motherboard
   c. Memory
   d. BIOS
5. What device runs the start-up instructions during boot-up of the computer?
   a. CPU
   b. Motherboard
   c. Memory
   d. BIOS
6. Random access memory will retain stored information after the computer has been shut down.
   a. True
   b. False
7. Which is considered the most versatile type of port found on a computer?
   a. Parallel
   b. USB
   c. IDE
   d. SCSI
8. The network card is designed to take the brunt of the force during a power surge.
   a. True
   b. False
9. Which of the following are types of computer mice?
   a. Infrared
   b. Mechanical
   c. Optical
   d. All of the above
10. Which type of monitor is most common in hospitals?
    a. OLED
    b. CRT
    c. LCD
    d. Plasma

Networking and Communication Basics

OBJECTIVES

On completion of this chapter, you should be able to:
- Distinguish between different types of networks (geographic and component roles).
- Identify common network hardware components.
- Describe different types of network cabling and their uses.
- Define *network protocol*.
- Differentiate between the common network topologies.
- Discuss the use of digital imaging and communications in medicine (DICOM) in medical imaging.
- Define *HL-7*, and describe its use in health care information systems.

OUTLINE

Network Classifications
    Geographic Classifications
    Component Role Classification
Typical Components of a Network
    Computers
    Network Connectivity
    Network Communication
Network Topology
    Bus
    Ring
    Star
    Mesh
Application Interfacing
    DICOM
    HL-7
Summary

KEY TERMS

Bus topology	Network router
Client-based network	Network switch
Coaxial cable	Peer-to-peer network
Digital imaging and communications in medicine (DICOM)	Radiology information system (RIS)
Fiber optic cable	Ring topology
HL-7	Server
Hospital information system (HIS)	Server-based network
Local area network (LAN)	Star topology
Mesh topology	Thick client
Network	Thin client
Network bridge	Topology
Network hub	Twisted-pair wire
Network interface card (NIC)	Wide area network (WAN)
Network protocol	Wireless
	Wireless access point

People use all types of networks every day to do things such as check the status of a package being shipped or register for a class at school. Many daily tasks involve transferring information, either from person to person (Figure 8-1) or from computer to computer (Figure 8-2).

A computer **network** is defined as (1) two or more objects sharing resources and information, or (2) computers, terminals, and servers that are interconnected by communication channels sharing data and program resources. Devices other than computers can also be found on a network, such as printers, scanners, and barcode readers. These devices can be shared among a group of computers to save money and space for the users.

This chapter explores network classifications, whether they are based on geographic boundaries or on the various roles that the hardware components play. An overview of the basic hardware components that make up a computer network and how the networks are physically constructed is also included. This chapter also provides a brief introduction to how medical devices, such as computed tomography (CT) scanners and computed radiography (CR) readers, fit within a network and how they communicate.

NETWORK CLASSIFICATIONS

Geographic Classifications

A network can be classified into two major geographic categories: local area network (LAN) and wide area network (WAN). (Other geographic classifications exist, such as metropolitan area network (MAN), tiny area network (TAN), and controller area network (CAN), but these are of little consequence to radiology.) These two terms

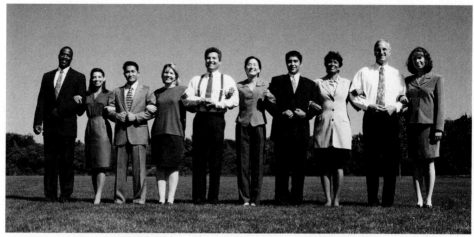

FIGURE 8-1 Person-to-person communication chain.

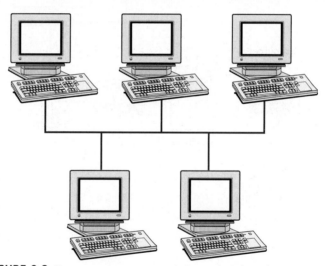

FIGURE 8-2 Five computers connected via a network to share resources.

are fairly self-explanatory: a LAN is close by, whereas a WAN expands over a distance.

Local Area Network. A local area network (LAN) (Figure 8-3) is a small area networked with a series of cables or **wireless access points** that allow computers to share information and devices on the same network. LANs are the least expensive to install, and they are much faster than WANs because of their smaller size. A LAN has the fastest communication technology because less equipment and fewer resources are needed to complete the network. Generally the larger networks are composed of several LANs interconnected to create the WAN. The picture archiving and communication system (PACS) workstations in a radiology reading room would be considered a LAN. The computers are interconnected and communicate by sharing images and reports.

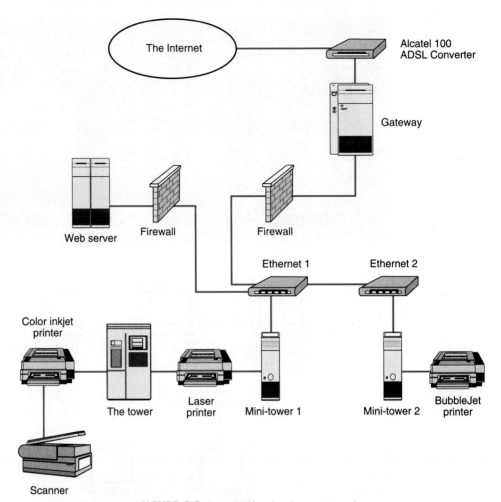

FIGURE 8-3 Typical office local area network.

Wide Area Network. A wide area network (WAN) is a network that spans a large area: city, state, nation, continent, or the world (Figure 8-4) It is used to connect computers that are not physically attached through conventional network cables but are rather connected through other means, such as telephone lines, satellite links, or other types of communication cable. The use of these long distance communication links drives up the operating costs of this type of network because most often these communication links are owned by a separate company, and because of the distance covered, the cost of having the highest speed equipment is expensive.

Component Role Classification

Networks are typically classified as either peer-to-peer or server/client-based, depending on what role their various components play. The network is classified according

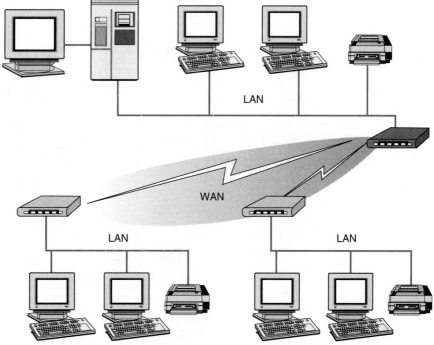

FIGURE 8-4 Wide area network (WAN) connecting several local area networks (LANs).

to what role the computers play in the network's operation and which computer controls the network operation.

Peer-to-Peer Network. In a **peer-to-peer network** (Figure 8-5), each computer on the network is considered equal; no computer has ultimate control over another. Each computer controls its own information and operation and can function either as a client or as a server depending on the needs of the other computers on the network. The peer-to-peer network is the most popular small office or home network configuration because it is the least expensive and most simple to set up. However, a peer-to-peer network has a limited scope because the maximum number of peers that should be connected is 10. More than 10 peers causes bottlenecks and collisions on the network. An example of a peer-to-peer network is a small medical office with several computers connected to check in patients, verify insurance, produce bills for the service, and document patient history. A printer is shared among the group of computers.

Server-Based Network. In a **server-based network** (Figure 8-6), there is a centralized computer (the server) that controls the operations, files, and sometimes the programs of the computers (the clients) attached to the network. The server provides a location for centralized storage and retrieval on the network. This allows the users to move from computer to computer and access their files from a central location. When a client requests a file, the server sends the entire file to the client for processing. Once the processing is completed, the client sends the entire changed file back to the server for storage. This type of network requires that the server be of high quality and high capacity, although the client computers can be less expensive.

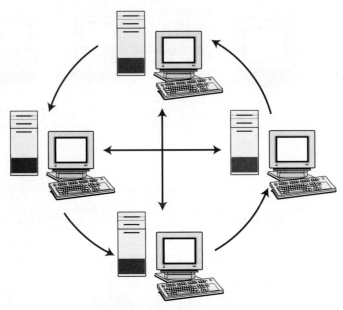

Resources are shared among
equals in a peer-to-peer network.

FIGURE 8-5 Peer-to-peer network.

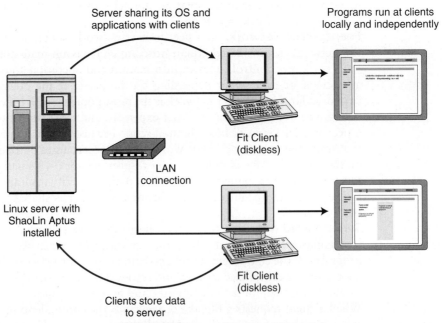

Server sharing its OS and
applications with clients

Programs run at clients
locally and independently

Fit Client
(diskless)

LAN
connection

Linux server with
ShaoLin Aptus
installed

Fit Client
(diskless)

Clients store data
to server

FIGURE 8-6 Server/client-based network.

There can be multiple servers on this type of network, but there must be one dedicated server that controls the network. An example of this type of network is a radiology department using a PACS to read and distribute images throughout the hospital. Computers throughout the hospital are connected to the centralized server that contains all of the images, and the images are sent out to the computers as requested.

Client-Based Network. A **client-based network** is similar to a server-based network in that there is a centralized computer that controls the operations of the network; however, rather than sending the entire original resource to the client for processing, the server processes the resource as requested by the client and returns only the results back to the client. This smaller exchange of information lessens the load on the network and allows more room for other requests.

TYPICAL COMPONENTS OF A NETWORK

Computers

Typically there are three types of computers found on a network: server, thin client, and thick client (Figure 8-7). Each of the three has a specific purpose on the network.

A **server** is a computer that manages resources for other computers, servers, and networked devices. It may also house applications, provide storage for files, or manage various other networked tasks. A server is most often dedicated to one task for the network and is usually the most robust computer on the network. There may be one server that provides storage for files, one that manages the print functions, and another that provides Internet access for the network.

A **thin client** is a device that is found on a network that requests services and resources from a server. The thin client may be another computer, a printer, or any other networkable device that needs a server to complete its tasks. Almost any personal computer (PC) can be a client, as long as it can be attached to the network.

A **thick client** is a computer that can work independently of the network and process and manage its own files. The thick client is networked so that it can share

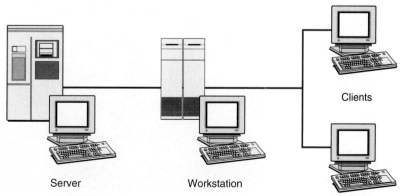

Clients

Server   Workstation

FIGURE 8-7 A server, workstation, and client on a network.

resources such as printing and take advantage of the additional security available on networks through dedicated servers. A thick client is generally a high-end computer that does high-level processing for specific purposes. In health care, specialty application workstations (thick client) are most often found in sectional imaging modalities for which three-dimensional (3D) imaging is used to aid diagnosis. The sectional images are fed into the workstation's application, and the application transforms the slices into a 3D image that can be evaluated.

Network Connectivity

Communication Medium. Once it has been determined what files and resources are to be shared and the pieces of equipment are in place, the components are connected via some sort of communication medium. The connection between the devices is one of four types: coaxial cable, twisted-pair wire, fiber optic cable, or electromagnetic waves. Several factors determine which type of communication medium is most appropriate.

Coaxial cable (Figure 8-8) is similar to the wiring used for the cable television that is run into a house. This type of cable consists of a center conducting wire surrounded by insulation and then a grounded shield of braided wire. The shield minimizes electrical and radio frequency interference. Coaxial cable is the sturdiest wire used and is often found in the network infrastructure throughout a building. It is often connected to another type of communication medium before it meets the device interface.

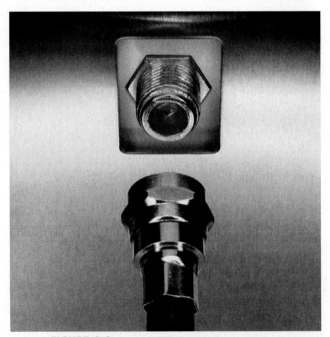

FIGURE 8-8 Coaxial cable network connection.

Twisted-pair wire (Figure 8-9) is similar to telephone wire, but whereas telephone wire has only four wires, twisted-pair wire usually consists of four twisted pairs of copper wires that are insulated and bundled together with an RJ-45 termination. Twisted-pair wire comes in various levels of quality and capacity. The minimum recommended standard is Cat 5 (category 5) cable. It is the most commonly used connection medium in LANs.

Fiber optic cable (Figure 8-10) uses glass threads to transmit data on the network. It consists of a fiber optic core that is surrounded by a plastic protective covering. This type of cable is much faster than its metal counterparts, but it is more expensive and much more fragile. Fiber optic cabling can easily be damaged by kinking and twisting the cable. It is most often used in the infrastructure of the network, in network closets, and in large archive/computer rooms.

Wireless connections (Figure 8-11) are becoming more commonplace as technology continues to improve. The connection is made by using either infrared or radio frequencies as its means of communication. There is no physical cabling needed, but each device must contain the appropriate wireless transmitter/receiver. The biggest advantage of wireless connections is mobility and convenience, but these kinds of connections have a limited range. When using wireless access points as the means of connection, the thickness and composition of the wall and the distance from the source must be taken into account.

Network Interface Card. The **network interface card** (**NIC**) (Figure 8-12) provides the interface between the computer and the network medium; it provides the physical connection between the network and computer. The NIC works with networking software to establish and manage the data, to chop up the data into packets, and to handle addressing issues. Most NICs plug directly into the motherboard as an expansion card, but they can also come as small adapter cards that insert into a slot on the side of the portable computer (Figure 8-13).

Network Hub. A **network hub** is the simplest device that can be used to connect several pieces of equipment together for network communication purposes. It has

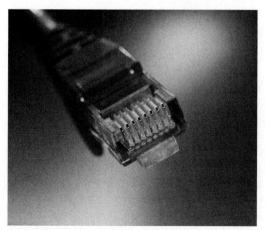

FIGURE 8-9 RJ-45 jack connected with twisted-pair Ethernet wire.

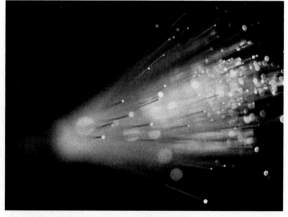

FIGURE 8-10 The glow from glass fibers in a fiber optic cable.

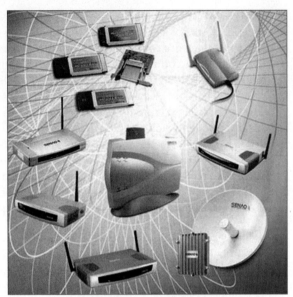

FIGURE 8-11 Wireless routers.

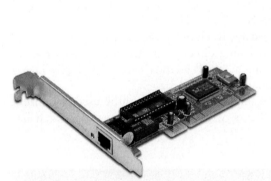

FIGURE 8-12 Network interface card (NIC).

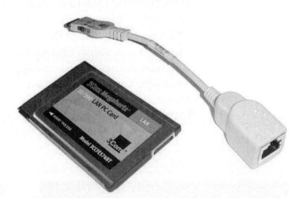

FIGURE 8-13 External NIC for a laptop computer.

several wiring ports available on it to receive and transmit data to the various connected pieces of equipment. When the hub receives data from a device, it generally sends those data to all devices connected to it. The hub does not know what the data are, nor to which device they should go, so it simply forwards the bits. Hubs are commonly used in small office and home applications.

Network Switch. A **network switch** is similar to a hub, but it sends data only to those devices to which the data are directed. It will read the destination address from the data and select a direct path to the intended target. This reduces the network traffic, speeds up the overall network connection, and makes the network more efficient. In general, switches are not commonly used in small office or home applications because there is not enough traffic to warrant the equipment.

Network Bridge. A **network bridge** is sometimes created so that larger networks can be segmented or broken up into smaller networks to reduce traffic within that network. These segments can then be connected with a bridge. The bridge is a physical (wired) connection from one network segment to another. It can recognize in which segment a particular destination address resides and send data to it. The bridge can also bring two or more networks together that speak the same language (i.e., use the same protocol).

Network Router. A **network router** is a more sophisticated device. It can read portions of messages and direct them to their intended target, even if the device is on a separate network and uses a different network protocol. It also helps with segmenting the network to allow access only for approved devices within that segment. In large networks there will be multiple routers, switches, and hubs that work in concert to perform the necessary tasks that enable the network to perform up to its potential.

Network Communication

We have learned that devices communicate via a NIC through some sort of communication medium. We know that the data are sent through some sort of box and that the box reads the destination address in the data to send them to the appropriate target. The question now is, Where does the address come from?

Each computer on the network is assigned a unique address. The address is a combination of a physical address from the computer's hardware and a node address given by the network. One type of addressing is Internet protocol (IP) addressing, which is made up of four octets (groups of 8 bits) of numbers. The numbers range from 0 to 255 (e.g., 144.162.21.107). The first set of numbers indicates the network class, and the rest of the numbers tell other devices the network's exact location. When a message is sent, the computer's NIC will read the destination address and check to see whether it matches the computer's network address. If it matches, it will receive the message. If it does not match, it just ignores the message.

The data travel along the network using an agreed-on set of rules known as a **network protocol**. Most network protocols send data in packets from one device to another. A packet is a piece of the data with added information, such as the destination address, the source address, the sequence of the packets (e.g., 2 of 12), and whether there were any errors in transmission. The protocol is delivered in layers of communication known as protocol stacks. Each layer of the communication represents a particular aspect of network functionality.

Typically a network communication model is explained using seven layers (OSI Model). We need to understand only the basic principles of network communication, so we will simplify the model and concentrate on the bottom four layers.

- Layer 4: The transport layer makes sure data packets are sequenced correctly and that they do not contain errors. For example, the most common transport-layer protocol, the transmission control protocol (TCP), resides in layer 4 and manages the connection for the purpose of controlling the flow of the data packets.
- Layer 3: The network layer breaks up the data into frames and decides which network path the frame will take to its destination. For example, the IP mentioned above is concerned with sending the message to the correct address.

- Layer 2: The data link layer packages the data so that they can be transmitted over the physical layer. Ethernet is an example protocol that performs at layer 2 and layer 1 levels.
- Layer 1: The physical layer consists of the networking media and the components required to pass on a signal from one end of the network to the other. This is the layer that moves bits from one place to another.

The most important thing to understand is that because of this standardized model, different types of networkable machines can be connected to transmit data to each other. As long as the machines share the same low-level protocols or know how to convert from one into another, the packets can be received and reconstructed.

NETWORK TOPOLOGY

Topology is the physical (geometric) layout of the connected devices on a network. There are four common topology configurations: bus, ring, star, and mesh. Many things should be considered when deciding what type of topology should be used, such as the type of communication media, the network speed, the connecting equipment design, and the number of devices to be connected. Each of these four is discussed in the following sections.

Bus

A **bus topology** (Figure 8-14) is a network in which all devices are physically attached to and listen for communication on a single wire. In a true bus network there is a single point of failure, the wire. If at some point on the wire there is a break, the entire network is down. (In some circumstances communication can take place between the computers on either side of the break.) This type of topology does not need any switches or hubs because the computers simply broadcast all the information down the single wire, and all computers connected to that single wire receive the information.

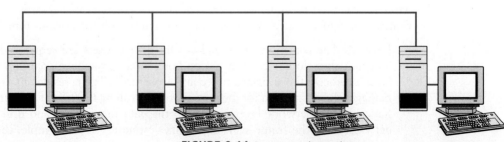

FIGURE 8-14 Bus network topology.

Ring

A **ring topology** (Figure 8-15) is a network in which the devices are connected in a circle. Each device passes its received messages to the next node on the ring (always in the same direction), and the data transmissions move around the circle until they reach the correct receiver. If there is a break at some point in the ring, the entire network comes to a halt.

One type of ring topology is called a token ring. The computers are connected in a circle, and a token is transmitted around the ring. When a computer is ready to send a transmission to another computer, it picks up the empty token as it passes by and fills it with the message. As the token passes the other computers, the destination address is read by each passing computer and is ignored if the address does not belong to that computer. When the addressed computer is found, the data are deposited, and the token is now free again. If another computer wishes to send out information but the token is occupied, it must wait until the token becomes free again before it can transmit.

Star

A **star topology** (Figure 8-16) is a network that has the devices connected to a central hub or switch. A star topology can be thought of as a bus topology with the bus collapsed into a central box: the hub or switch. The data are sent through the hub out to the destination device. This transmission of data may be through another hub or switch to an adjacent network or directly to the device. Star topology is the most commonly used network topology.

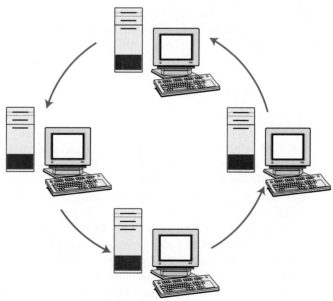

FIGURE 8-15 Ring network topology.

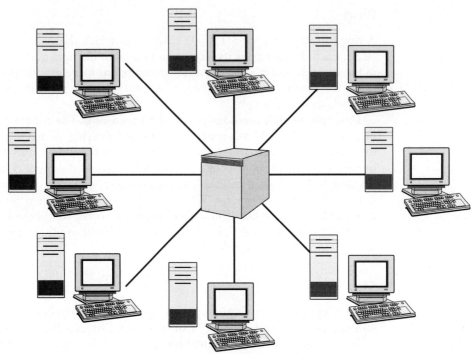

FIGURE 8-16 Star network topology.

Mesh

A **mesh topology** (Figure 8-17) is a network that has multiple pathways interconnecting devices and networks. This type of network has redundancy built in with the multiple connections. The Internet is based on mesh topology, and this topology is used most often to connect networks to other networks.

APPLICATION INTERFACING

DICOM

DICOM, which stands for **d**igital **i**maging and **co**mmunications in **m**edicine, has become an almost universally accepted standard for exchanging medical images among networked medical devices. DICOM is layered on top of TCP/IP, the most common network communication standard used, and it has multiple layers as does TCP/IP.

DICOM was developed by the American College of Radiology (ACR) and the National Electrical Manufacturers Association (NEMA). The first version was completed in 1985, addressing only point-to-point connections between devices. At publication of this book, the current version is 3-2011. (There are revisions and additions always in progress.) Up-to-date information can be found on NEMA's website at http://medical.nema.org.

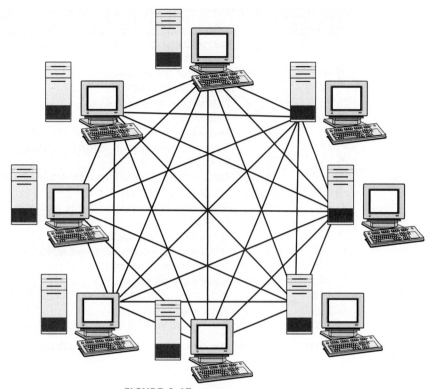

FIGURE 8-17 Mesh network topology.

DICOM (3.0) is better than its predecessors for several reasons:

- It required a communications protocol that runs on top of TCP/IP (or other standardized protocol stack), permitting the devices to make use of commercial hardware and software.
- It required strict contents of the image "header" and the structure of the pixel data itself for each type of modality, therefore improving interoperability.
- It required a conformance system, so that a user could determine from the vendor's documentation whether the devices would operate together.
- It embraced an open standard of development between the vendors and users to come to consensus on the direction of the standards.

The DICOM standard is made up of 20 different parts ranging from image display to media storage. Not every device conforms to every part of the DICOM, but rather a device will conform to the parts that are necessary to perform the tasks it is assigned according to what is desired by the user. The standard is maintained on a continuous basis and is published periodically. Supplements are published with new updates and error corrections, and new parts are being investigated as new functions are developed. Table 8-1 lists the 20 parts of the DICOM standard and their corresponding titles.

The DICOM standard defines so-called service classes or functions that a device can perform on a defined information object (such as a CT image). The allowed

TABLE 8-1	The 20 Parts of the DICOM Standard 3-2011
PS 3.1	Introduction and overview
PS 3.2	Conformance
PS 3.3	Information object definitions
PS 3.4	Service class specifications
PS 3.5	Data structures and encoding
PS 3.6	Data dictionary
PS 3.7	Message exchange
PS 3.8	Network communication support for message exchange
PS 3.9	Retired
PS 3.10	Media storage and file format for media interchange
PS 3.11	Media storage application profiles
PS 3.12	Media formats and physical media for media interchange
PS 3.13	Retired
PS 3.14	Grayscale standard display function
PS 3.15	Security and system management profiles
PS 3.16	Content mapping resource
PS 3.17	Explanatory information
PS 3.18	Web access to DICOM-persistent objects (WADO)
PS 3.19	Application hosting
PS 3.20	Transformation of DICOM to and from HL-7 Standards

DICOM, Digital imaging and communications in medicine; *HL-7*, Health Level 7.

service/object pairs (SOPs) for a device are spelled out explicitly in the device's DICOM conformance statement. A device performs either as a service class user (SCU) for a given service and object or as a service class provider (SCP) or as both. The SCU and SCP are commonly referred to as roles. Network communications (i.e., transactions) in DICOM are always between an SCP and an SCU. The following are the most common service classes seen in modalities and PACS:

- Image storage
- Query/retrieval
- Print
- Modality worklist
- Modality performed procedure
- Storage commitment
- Interchange media storage

Each of these services defines a specific transaction for the modality and PACS, and because of the standardization provided by DICOM, device interoperability is possible (or at least more likely). The DICOM conformance statement of a device details the various SOPs and possible roles that the modality or workstation can fulfill with those SOPs. For example, if a magnetic resonance imaging (MRI) scanner conformance statement lists the MRI storage SOP class in the SCU role, and the receiving PACS archive lists MRI storage SOP class in the SCP role, the MRI scanner would be able to send images to the archive based on those statements. If either statement does not support the proper SOP class and role, the transfer is not possible. Most modalities manufactured today are DICOM conformant. The vendors will provide conformance statements, and the buyer must closely inspect these statements to ensure that the modalities can communicate with existing image viewing devices.

DICOM also has specifications for uniquely identifying each study, series, and image (instance). DICOM uses unique identifiers (UIDs) to globally identify each image set, so that if the images are sent to multiple systems, the identifying number will remain unique and not be confused with those images on other systems. Each study is identified by a study instance UID, which breaks down into series instance UIDs, and further into instance UIDs. The numbers are created based on a vendor number, serial number of the equipment, date, time, patient or processing number, and then the study, series, or image number. A typical study instance UID may look like this: 1.2.840.8573.4567.1.20051011764589.8765.1.

DICOM also provides a framework for the use of compression technologies on image data. For example, DICOM accommodates joint photographic experts group (JPEG) lossless compression of 2 to 1. This is the most common compression technique used within hospitals because there is no image degradation on viewing after decompression. But when moving images outside of the hospital, it may be necessary to use lossy compression to shrink the file size to suit external networks. Some loss of image detail can occur when higher compression values are used.

When a patient arrives for a procedure, the technologist either has to manually type in the patient's demographics, risking error, or alternatively pull the information directly from the radiology information system (RIS). A modality can pull this information when it supports the service class of modality worklist management, and the RIS can either interface via DICOM or through a gateway that creates an interface with the Health Level 7 (HL-7) device and the DICOM device.

After an image has been captured, all of the demographic information and information about the actual capture of the image is recorded in the image header. The DICOM image header contains many different elements, such as the patient name, ID, referring physician, the number of images in the study, and it can also contain the actual technical factors used for the capture. In digital projection radiography, the kilovoltage peak (kVp), milliampere-seconds (mAs), and the exposure indices are captured on all but cassette-based storage phosphor systems. The technologist must realize that any manipulation of an image will be recorded in this header and he or she is held legally responsible for any image manipulation that occurs.

HL-7

HL-7 is an American National Standards Institute (ANSI)–accredited Standards Developing Organization (SDO).

The standards set by this organization are used in most health care applications such as medical devices, imaging, insurance, and pharmacy. The HL-7 standards oversee most clinical and administrative data such as demographics, reports, claims, and orders. As with DICOM, HL-7 is composed of many parts and is used at many levels within various hospital systems. HL-7 standards are generally used in communication between the **hospital information system (HIS)** and the **radiology** information system (RIS). The HIS holds the patient's full medical information, from hospital billing to the inpatient ordering system. The RIS holds all radiology-specific patient data, from the patient scheduling information to the radiologist's dictated and transcribed report. The electronic medical record (EMR) has recently come to the forefront of information technology. The EMR is either a part of the HIS or runs along with it and contains all of the patient's record, including lab results, radiology reports, pathology results, and nurses' and doctors' notes. The EMR interfaces with most of the ancillary service systems to retrieve reports so that they can be viewed in this one common format. PACS have also begun interfacing with EMRs to present images to referring physicians through the same common system.

SUMMARY

- A network is defined as two or more objects sharing resources and information.
- A network can be classified into two major geographic categories: local area network (LAN) and wide area network (WAN). There are two typical classifications of networks based on the roles that various components play: peer-to-peer and server/client-based.
- A server is a computer that manages resources for other computers, servers, and networked devices. A client is a device that is found on a network that requests services and resources from a server. A thick client is a computer that can work independently of the network and can process and manage its own files. A thin client server depends on another computer that serves as the data processor for the bulk of information.
- The connection among the devices is one of the following four types: coaxial cable, twisted-pair wire, fiber optic cable, or electromagnetic waves.
- Information is transmitted via a network interface card (NIC) through a communication medium onto the network and possibly through a hub, switch, bridge, or router.
- The data travel along the network using an agreed-on set of rules known as a protocol.
- Topology is the physical layout of the connected devices on a network. There are four common topologic configurations: bus, ring, star, and mesh.
- DICOM stands for digital imaging and communications in medicine. It is a universally accepted standard for exchanging medical images among networked medical devices.
- DICOM defines specific information objects and the functions (service classes) that can be performed on them.
- The HL-7 standard oversees most clinical and administrative data such as demographics, reports, claims, and orders.
- The HIS holds the patient's full medical information, from hospital billing to the inpatient ordering system. The RIS holds all radiology-specific patient data, from the patient scheduling information to the radiologist's dictated and transcribed report.

CHAPTER REVIEW QUESTIONS

1. Which of the following are network classifications based on geographic location?
   a. LAN
   b. WAN
   c. MAN
   d. All of the above

2. On a server-based network, each computer is considered equal.
   a. True
   b. False

3. In which type of network does a centralized computer have control over the entire network?
   a. Peer-to-peer
   b. Server-based
   c. Client-based
   d. Both b & c

4. Which of the following types of computer found on a network can work independently of the network and process/manage its own files but still share printing and storage?
   a. Thin client
   b. Thick client
   c. Server
   d. All of the above

5. Which of the following network communication medium has a single conductive wire surrounded by a grounded shield of braided wire?
   a. Coaxial cable
   b. Twisted-pair wire
   c. Fiber optic cable
   d. Ethernet

6. Which of the following is the most delicate network communication medium?
   a. Coaxial cable
   b. Twisted pair wire
   c. Fiber optic cable
   d. Ethernet

7. What provides the interface between the computer and the network medium?
   a. Network hub
   b. Network switch
   c. Network interface card
   d. Network router

8. What is the simplest network hardware device that can be used to connect several computers?
   a. Network hub
   b. Network switch
   c. Network interface card
   d. Network router

9. What is an agreed-upon set of rules that data use to move through a network?
   a. Topology
   b. Network protocol
   c. Mesh
   d. NIC
10. Which of the following is used to move medical images from the modality to the viewing/storage device?
   a. NEMA
   b. HL-7
   c. DICOM
   d. ANSI

PACS Fundamentals

OBJECTIVES

On completion of this chapter, you should be able to:
- Define *picture archiving and communication system (PACS)*.
- Compare and contrast the various types of PACS display workstations.
- Differentiate among the different types of digital imaging work flow.
- Define *system architecture* and recognize the three major models.
- Summarize the common functions found on a PACS workstation.
- Describe the situations and users that may require advanced PACS workstation functions.

The **picture archiving and communication system (PACS)** is becoming more commonplace in today's hospitals because hospital administrators have come to see the necessity of having such a system to serve physicians and patients even though it is expensive. The initial capital cost is great, but the benefit of having the system far outweighs the cost. This chapter outlines the basic concept of a PACS and its components, describes common PACS architecture, and gives examples of typical PACS work flows that may be seen in a hospital.

FUNDAMENTALS

As discussed in Chapter 1, a PACS consists of digital acquisition, display workstations, and storage devices interconnected through an intricate network (Figure 9-1). The PACS is an electronic version of the radiologist reading room and the file room. The first PACSs were used in the early 1980s and generally served a single modality. Large research institutions housed early systems because most were developed by the scientists who worked at those institutions. As vendors became more involved, they developed proprietary systems that were very specific to their modalities. Finally, as physicians and hospitals became interested, it was determined that there must be standardization.

Digital imaging and communications in medicine (DICOM) is a universally accepted standard for exchanging medical images among the modality, viewing stations, and the archive. First completed in 1985, this standard laid the groundwork for the future development of integrated PACSs. Now each modality and PACS communicates via DICOM, and DICOM continues to be refined every year. Every vendor and modality boasts DICOM compatibility (Figure 9-2), but each DICOM statement must be read carefully to determine the extent of the compatibility. DICOM compatibility issues are outside of the scope of this textbook.

To understand what a PACS is and how it is used, it helps to look at the system's individual parts. The following sections break down a PACS into its three fundamental parts (Figure 9-3): image acquisition, display workstations, and archive servers. Each of these topics is covered in depth in other chapters of the book.

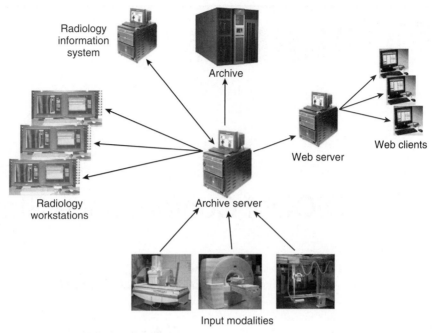

FIGURE 9-1 A typical PACS design.

Image Acquisition

In modern radiology departments, most images are acquired in a digital format, meaning that the images are inherently digital and can be transferred via a computer network. Ultrasound, computed tomography (CT), magnetic resonance imaging (MRI), and nuclear medicine have been digital for many years and have been taking advantage of PACS far longer than general radiography has. As stated earlier, the first PACS served a single modality, namely, ultrasound. Ultrasound mini-PACS networks were the norm in many hospitals. Radiologists routinely made diagnoses by looking at images on the modality's computer screen. It was a natural step from there to convert ultrasound to **softcopy** reporting (i.e., reading images on the computer without hardcopy films).

As the CT and MRI image sets became larger because of the increased number of cross-sectional images per patient, radiologists routinely went to the modality to view the images. This slowed down the scanning process for the technologists, and vendors began getting requests for extra console stations for radiologist viewing. These workstations were directly connected to the modalities. Radiologists could view the large stacks of images and perform simple image manipulation. These workstations morphed into mini-PACS and eventually into full-blown systems for CT and MRI. As discussed in Chapters 4 through 7, general radiography has taken the digital leap with digital projection radiography. Now the conversion to a completely digital radiology department is a reality.

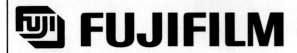

DICOM Conformance Statement

CR Console

(Standard)

April, 2004
5th Edition

FIGURE 9-2 A DICOM conformance statement for a CT scanner. *(Courtesy FUJIFILM Medical Systems USA, Inc.)*

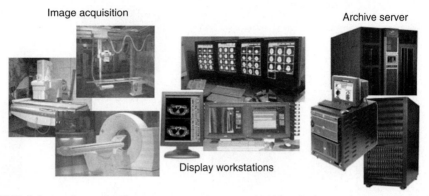

FIGURE 9-3 A collage of PACS components: image acquisition, display workstation, and archive server.

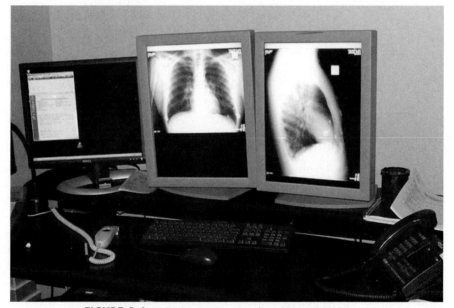

FIGURE 9-4 A display workstation for image review.

Display Workstations

A **display workstation** is any computer that a health care worker uses to view a digital image (Figure 9-4). It is the most interactive part of a PACS, and these workstations are used inside and outside of radiology. The display station receives images from the archive or from the various radiology modalities and presents them for viewing. The display workstation has PACS application software that allows the user to perform minor image-manipulation techniques to optimize the image being viewed. Some display stations have advanced software to perform more complex image-manipulation techniques. More details about display workstations are given later in the chapter.

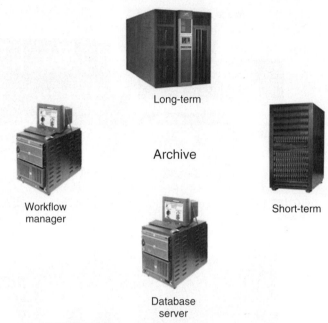

Long-term

Archive

Workflow
manager

Short-term

Database
server

FIGURE 9-5 The common components of an archive.

Archive Servers

An archive server is the file room of the PACS. It is composed of a database server or image manager, short-term and long-term storage, and a computer that controls the PACS workflow, known as a workflow manager (Figure 9-5). The archive is the central part of the PACS and houses all of the historic data along with the current data being generated. In many institutions the archive serves as the central hub that receives all images before they are released to the radiologists for interpretation. The archive and all of its components are studied in depth in Chapter 10.

Workflow

Workflow is a term that can be used in any industry or in any organization. It simply means how a process is done, step by step. In radiology, the term *workflow* has always been used to describe how an examination is completed, from order entry to transcribed report. This section describes a generic film-based workflow and then compares it with a generic PACS workflow. The workflow in each radiology department is different because there are many variables.

Film-Based Workflow. Most departments were designed years ago for film and chemical processing. Pass boxes were built into walls that fed into darkrooms and into large open reading rooms that had gigantic multiviewer lightboxes lining the walls (see Figure 9-11). Eventually chemical-processing time decreased from a few minutes to less than 60 seconds in some cases. As film and processing technology advanced, workflow became more efficient, despite the fact that technologists still

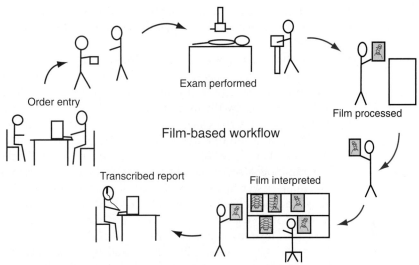

Exam performed

Order entry

Film-based workflow

Film processed

Transcribed report

Film interpreted

FIGURE 9-6 A typical film-based workflow from order entry to transcribed report.

have to hand-deliver film to radiologists and make the occasional copy for a referring physician.

The following list outlines a typical workflow in a radiology department, from entering the order to transcribing the report (Figure 9-6).

- The first step in any radiology department workflow is the entry of the order. The order may be a paper prescription from the ordering doctor, or the order may have been placed in the computer system by any hospital staff member. Either way, an order is placed in the radiology information system (RIS), and a requisition is generated. A requisition generally contains the following information:
  - Patient's name
  - Patient's hospital identification (ID) number
  - Date of birth
  - Ordering physician's name
  - Examination ordered
  - Reason for examination
  - Chief complaint
- The paper requisition is then passed on to the technologist who will be performing the examination.
- The technologist prepares the room for the patient and brings the patient back to the room.
- The technologist verifies all of the patient's information and completes a patient history. The technologist also inquires whether the patient needs a complete set of copies to take to the next doctor's appointment.
- The technologist performs the examination and processes all of the film after the complete examination is done.

- The technologist critiques each film and repeats exposures as necessary.
- The technologist makes copies if necessary and releases the patient with the copies.
- The technologist goes to the file room to find the film jacket with all of the patient's historic images, if applicable. The film jacket may not be located on site and may be kept at an off-site storage location. The film jacket is ordered to be picked up by the film courier.
- The film jacket arrives a couple of hours or even days later, and the current films are hung on a multiviewer lightbox to be read by a radiologist. The file room clerk may hang a set of historic images from the film jacket for comparison.
- The radiologist reads the films and dictates a report into the dictation system.
- The multiviewer lightbox is cleared of read films by the file room clerk, and the films are placed back into the film jacket. The film jacket is filed in the file room.
- A transcriptionist retrieves the recorded dictation and transcribes a report into the RIS. This may occur later that same day or the next day.
- The radiologist reviews the report, makes corrections, and signs the report as final. The final report is printed and placed in the patient's film jacket along with any previous reports. A final report is also sent to the ordering physician for review. This final report may come several days after the examination was completed.

Generic PACS Workflow. The PACS workflow is in many ways different from the film-based workflow (Figure 9-7). The technologist may get the order via an electronic worklist or a paper requisition, but after that, the process begins to change.

- Changes in the order entry are on the horizon, but for now, the order-entry process is the same as in film-based departments. The technologist needs a requisition to verify the patient ID and to take a patient history.

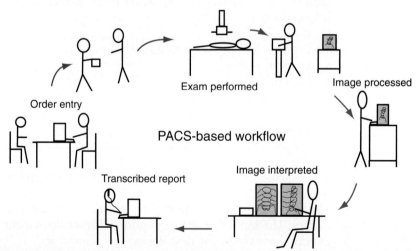

Exam performed

Image processed

Order entry

PACS-based workflow

Image interpreted

Transcribed report

FIGURE 9-7 This diagram represents a typical PACS-based workflow from order entry to transcribed report.

- The order is input into the RIS, and the RIS sends a message to the PACS to find all historic images and put them on the short-term archive. This eliminates waiting for the file room to retrieve a film jacket from the off-site storage location.
- The technologist prepares the room, retrieves the patient, and performs the patient history. The history is recorded on the paper requisition or input electronically into the patient's computerized medical record.
- The technologist performs the examination, and depending on the type of image acquisition device, the images are processed and repeated as necessary and sent to the appropriate PACS device. The patient images have been tagged with information from the RIS so that historic image reports are available at the PACS when the new images are sent. If the patient's physician does not have access to the electronic images, a compact disk (CD) or digital versatile disk (DVD) can be made that contains the images in digital format.
- The requisition is either taken to the radiologist, or the radiologist may pull the images from an electronic worklist. The radiologist also pulls up historic images and reports and compares the previous images with the current images.
- The radiologist dictates a report and has it transcribed, or voice recognition software may be used. If the radiologist uses voice recognition software, he or she can review the report right after dictation, make corrections, and sign the report, making it final.

With PACS it is possible that the time it takes from performing the examination to completing the final radiologist's report is only a couple of hours, compared with a couple of days for the film-based workflow.

SYSTEM ARCHITECTURE

System architecture can be defined as the hardware and software infrastructure of a computer system. In a PACS, the system architecture normally consists of acquisition devices, storage, display workstations, and an image management system. The following discussion outlines three common PACS architectures and takes a look at the flow of images after acquisition.

Client/Server-Based Systems

In a **client/server-based system**, images are sent directly to the archive server after acquisition and are centrally located (Figure 9-8). The display workstation functions as a client of the archive server and accesses images based on a centralized worklist that is generated at the archive server. The health care worker at the display workstation chooses a name from the central list, and the archive server sends the image data to the display station. After the "client" is finished, the image data are flushed from its memory. Most systems allow basic image manipulation at the display workstation or "client," and the changes are saved on the archive server.

Advantages
- Any examination sent to the PACS is available anywhere without other interventions.

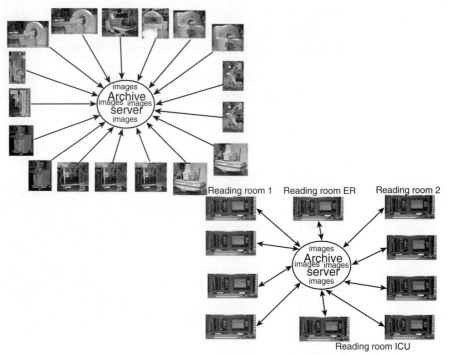

FIGURE 9-8 A client/server-based system architecture.

- Only one person can open the study with the intent to read it. Others that open the study will receive a message that the study is open and being read.
- There is no need to pull or send historic images to a particular workstation because the old studies are available with the new on the archive.

Disadvantages

- The archive server is seen as a single point of failure. If the archive goes down, the entire system is down, and no image movement can take place. All newly acquired images must remain at the modality until the archive is up and can again receive the images.
- The system is very network dependent. The images are flying back and forth between the archive and the workstations, and the network can become bogged down because of the large volume of data being moved.
- The archive server is handling many requests at once and can become bottle-necked because of the high volume of requests.

Distributed Systems

In a **distributed or stand-alone system,** the acquisition modalities send the images to a designated reading station and possibly to review stations, depending on where the order originated (i.e., the intensive care unit or the emergency room) (Figure 9-9). In some systems, the images are sent from the modality to the archive server, and the archive server distributes the images to the designated workstation. The reading station designations may be designed based on radiologist reading

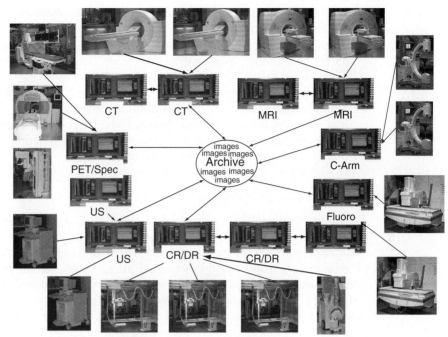

FIGURE 9-9 A distributed system architecture model.

preferences. For example, MRI may be sent to one station and CT to another, or all cross-sectional neurologic images may be sent to one station, but all body images are sent to another. The designation is decided after extensive workflow observation. Moreover, in a distributed model, the workstations can query and retrieve images from the archive. All images are then stored locally and subsequently sent to the archive server after they have been read. These images remain on the local hard drive of the workstation until they are deleted either by a user or at a predetermined time set by system rules.

Advantages
- If the archive server goes down, local reading at the workstations is not interrupted, other than not being able to get historic images. After the archive comes back up, the images that have been changed and signed off by the radiologist will be forwarded automatically to the archive to be saved.
- Because the images can be distributed to many locations at once, copies of an examination exist at various locations. Therefore it is less likely that PACS data will be lost.
- The system is less dependent on the network for its speed. The user can be working on one examination while the workstation is pulling and getting the next examination ready to be read. The workstation can fetch historic images according to rules the user sets up.

Disadvantages
- There is heavy reliance on the assumption that the distribution of images is being done correctly. If the distribution is wrong, the prefetching of historic examinations will not be correct either.

- Each workstation has a different worklist, and therefore only one person can be working on that list at a time.
- It can be inconvenient to read additional studies; the radiologist would have to move to another workstation to read the images designated for that workstation.
- The users must depend on the query-and-retrieve function when nonscheduled examinations arrive at the workstation to be read.
- It is also possible for two radiologists to be reading the same examination and not know that the other has it until they try to start dictation. The paper requisition is very important with this type of PACS.

Web-Based Systems

A **web-based system** is very similar to a client/server system in how data flow. The significant difference is that both the images and the application software for the client display are held centrally (Figure 9-10). This means that when someone wants to view images from a web-based application, he or she simply searches for the pertinent images and the web browser will display the images that are held in the web server. This does not require special software to be downloaded to the computer. In a client/server system, the application software is locally loaded to the client, and only the images are held at the archive.

Advantages
- The hardware at the client can be anything that will support an appropriate web browser. This allows for greater flexibility with hardware but can also be a disadvantage because image displays (monitors) may not be able to support diagnostic quality.
- The same application can be used on site and at home in teleradiology situations. Teleradiology is a term used to describe the reading of images from outside of

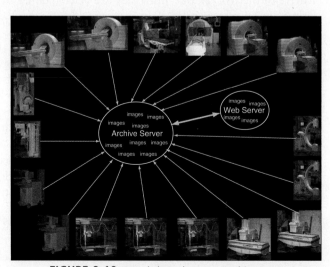

FIGURE 9-10 A web-based system architecture.

the hospital's walls. It can be down the road at the radiologist's home or on the other side of the world during nighttime hours. Many companies have been created over the past decade to provide these teleradiology services.

Disadvantages

- The system's functionality may be limited because the software is not installed locally. The bandwidth of the network connection limits the amount of data that can be transmitted for download, and some programs are too large to be transmitted over the network that is installed.
- As with client/server systems, in a web-based system the network is the biggest obstacle to performance.

DISPLAY WORKSTATIONS

The display workstation is the most interactive part of a PACS, consisting of a monitor and a computer with a mouse and keyboard. In addition, each system has hardware and software that fits the users' requirements.

As the technologist knows, conventional film/screen radiography uses large multiviewer lightboxes to display the images (Figure 9-11). Early in the history of PACSs, radiologists believed that they needed four to six monitors to match the viewing capability they had with the lightboxes. As the radiologists have become more comfortable viewing images on monitors, the number of monitors required

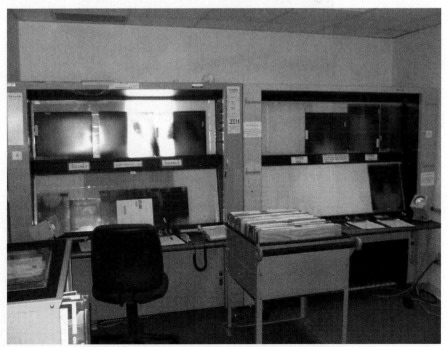

FIGURE 9-11 Multiviewer lightbox that was commonly seen in radiology departments for film viewing.

by the radiologists has decreased to an average of two (Figure 9-12). This decrease can also be attributed in part to the continued development of viewing software and better hardware, namely, mice.

The monitor is one of the most important elements of a PACS display station. The cathode ray tube (CRT) (Figure 9-13) and the liquid crystal display (LCD) (Figure 9-14) are the most popular types of monitors in a radiology department. The LCD has decreased in price and increased in quality and has taken over the entire PACS display market because of its size, resolution, and lack of heat production. The LCD also requires less maintenance, gives out more light, and can be used in areas with a high amount of ambient light. In early PACS reading rooms, supplemental air conditioning had to be installed to offset the heat put out by multiple CRTs. Along with the number of monitors used, the resolution and orientation of the monitor are also factors in determining which type of monitor to buy for each workstation. Most cross-sectional imaging is read on a 1K square monitor (Figure

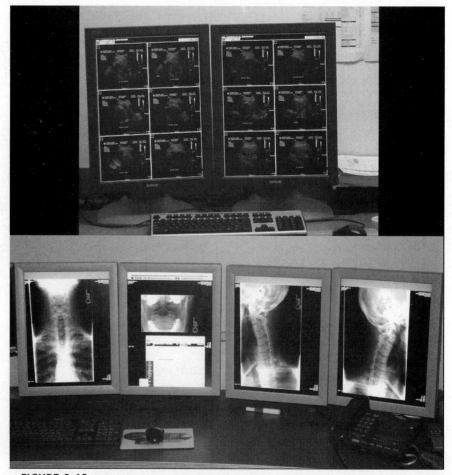

FIGURE 9-12 A four-bank monitor workstation and a two-bank monitor workstation.

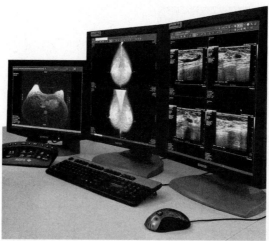

FIGURE 9-13 A cathode ray tube (CRT) monitor. *(Courtesy Agfa.)*

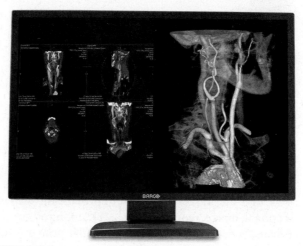

FIGURE 9-14 A liquid crystal display (LCD) monitor. *(Courtesy Barco.)*

9-15), and most digital projection images are read on at least a 2K portrait monitor (Figure 9-16).

Remember from Chapter 2 that a basic picture element on a display is known as a pixel. The number of pixels contained on a display is known as its resolution. The relationship between pixels and resolution can be stated as follows: the more pixels in an image, the higher the resolution of the image, and the more information that can be displayed. Resolution can also be defined as the process or capability of distinguishing between individual parts of an image that are adjacent. Pixels are arranged in a matrix. A matrix is a rectangular or square table of numbers that represents the pixel intensity to be displayed on the monitor. Common screen resolutions that are found on today's monitors are 1280×1024 (1K), 1600×1200 (2K), 2048×1536 (3K), and 2048×2560 (5K).

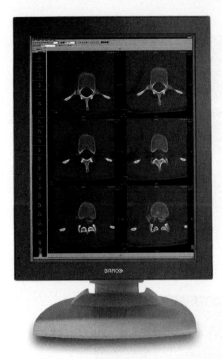

FIGURE 9-15 A 1K monitor. *(Courtesy Barco.)*

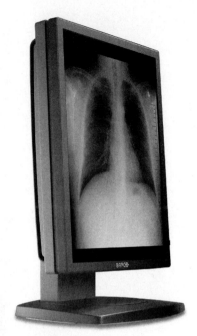

FIGURE 9-16 A 2K monitor. *(Courtesy Barco.)*

Medical display monitors are generally of a higher quality than display monitors used for other applications. Radiologists often use the highest resolution monitors available for the modality that is being read. For example, mammography requires a 5K or 5-megapixel resolution to provide the viewing capacity needed, but a cross-sectional image requires only a 1K monitor to view the necessary information. Because a referring physician is not the primary doctor reading the examinations, a 1K monitor would be sufficient for his or her viewing needs.

Display stations can be categorized by their primary use: primary reading stations for radiologists, review stations for referring physicians, technologist quality control (QC) stations where technologists review images, and image management stations for the file room personnel. Each of these workstations has one specific main purpose and is strategically located near the end user of its designated purpose.

Radiologist Reading Stations

The radiologist **reading station** (Figure 9-17) is used by a radiologist when making a primary diagnosis. The reading station has the highest quality hardware, including the best monitor. The computer hardware meets the needs of the PACS vendor, but it will usually be very robust, requiring little downtime. The keyboard and mouse can be customized. There are many different styles of mice available that can increase the efficiency of the software being used (Figure 9-18).

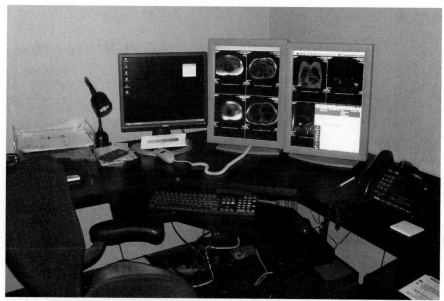

FIGURE 9-17 A radiologist reading station.

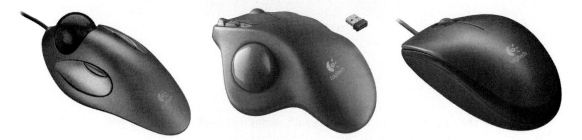

FIGURE 9-18 A wheel mouse, a trackball mouse, and an ergonomic mouse. *(Courtesy Logitech.)*

There is generally access to a nearby RIS, with a dictation system near or even connected to the PACS station. Many PACSs have software that integrates the RIS and dictation system.

Physician Review Stations

The physician **review workstation** (Figure 9-19) is a step-down model of the radiologist reading station. Many vendors use the same level of software but may eliminate some of the more advanced functions. One of the most important features on a physician review station is the ability to view current and previous reports along with the images. This can be accomplished with the integration of RIS functions with the PACS software mentioned above. Most referring physicians want to read

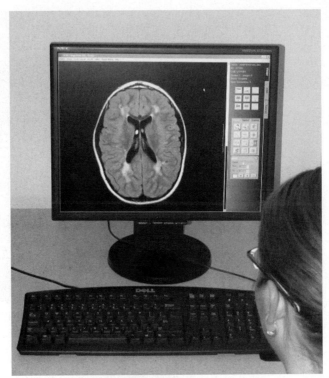

FIGURE 9-19 A physician review station.

the radiologist's report along with seeing the patient's images, and often the report is more important to them than the images.

The software may either be loaded on a stand-alone station that is dedicated to viewing images, or it may be delivered over a web browser on any personal computer (PC) within an office or on a floor. In high-volume areas such as the emergency room and the intensive care unit, there are dedicated PACS workstations for image viewing (Figure 9-20). These dedicated stations may have the higher-end monitors such as the radiologist reading stations, but many may have lower-end monitors because of cost constraints.

One of the greatest advantages of a PACS is the ability to view the same set of images in multiple locations at one time. In the film/screen era, referring physicians would make the trek to the radiology department to consult with a radiologist about a patient's image, hoping that the films would be found in the file room and that the radiologist was available to consult. Now with PACS, the referring physician can pull up the patient's images in his or her office and read the radiologist's report. The referring physician and the radiologist can consult on the telephone while looking at the images simultaneously. This is one way that PACSs have improved continuity and speed of patient care.

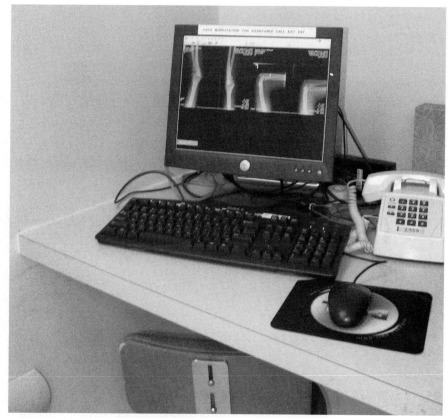

FIGURE 9-20 A physician review workstation.

Technologist QC Stations

The technologist **quality control (QC) station** (Figure 9-21) is used to review images after acquisition but before sending them to the radiologist. The QC station may be used to improve or adjust image quality characteristics, or it may be used to verify patient demographic information. Many QC stations are placed between the computed radiography (CR) and digital radiography (DR) acquisition modalities as a pass-through to ensure that the images have met the departmental quality standard. The technologist QC station generally has a 1K monitor. When manipulating images, the technologist must be careful not to change the appearance too much from the original acquired image. The technologist should consult frequently with the radiologist to ensure that the images being sent are of the required quality.

The QC workstation can also be used to query and retrieve historic images before beginning of an examination so that the technologist can check previous pathology or body characteristics. This can help with the selection of technical factors or procedural protocol. It is common protocol in a film-based department to pull film jackets on patients before performing an examination. The QC station affords the same benefit as pulling the film jacket.

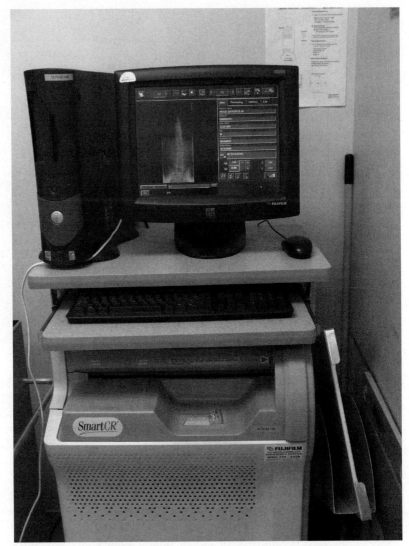

FIGURE 9-21 A technologist QC workstation.

File Room/Image Management Stations

The file room in a radiology department has seen many changes over the years. Before PACS, the file room was a large open room with endless rows of shelves full of film jackets. Today a file room in a PACS environment may be as simple as a couple of computers with CD/DVD burners and a dry laser to make copies for outside needs.

The **file room workstation** (Figure 9-22) may be used to look up examinations for a physician or to print copies of images for the patient to take to an outside physician. Many hospitals are moving away from printing films to save the cost of the film and are instead moving toward burning CDs with the patient's images

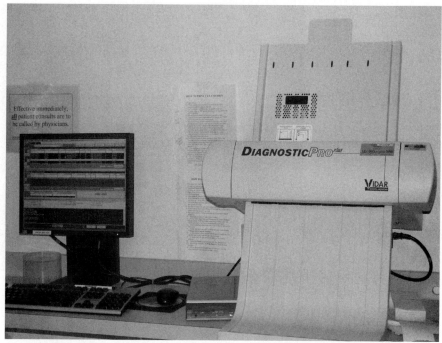

FIGURE 9-22 A file room workstation used for image management purposes.

because they are less expensive. The CD of images can be viewed on any PC and generally comes with easy-to-use software burned onto it with the images.

The file room personnel may also be responsible for correcting patient demographics. If images with incorrect demographics are sent to the archive, then it is difficult to pull those images the next time the patient comes in for an examination. The archive is a database and is only as good as the information that is put into it.

Common Functions

This section provides an overview of common functions found on a PACS workstation. All of the functions should be available on any level of the workstation except for the advanced functions, which are specific to different types of workstations. The functions can be broken down into four categories: navigation functions, image manipulation and enhancement functions, image management functions, and advanced workstation functions.

Navigation Functions. Navigation functions (Figure 9-23) are used to move through images, series, studies, and patients. The worklist is used to navigate through patients. Most worklists are customizable for the user. One doctor may want to see only unread CT studies, and another may want to see all neurologic studies done that day regardless of the modality. Most modern PACS software conforms to the Windows (Microsoft, Redmond, WA) look and feel. The use of grab bars on the right side of Windows to scroll through a list and the activation

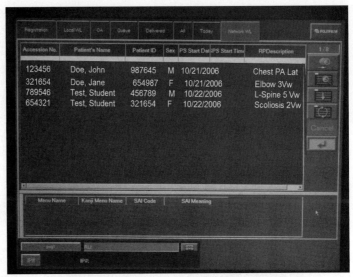

FIGURE 9-23 A screen shot of a PACS worklist.

of the scroll wheel on the mouse to scroll through the list are common features. The mouse is also a very useful navigation tool. The right mouse offers many shortcut features in a menu of frequently used tasks and applications.

Hanging Protocols. Once a patient has been selected from the worklist, the images load into the display software. In most PACSs, each user has the ability to set up custom hanging protocols. A **hanging protocol** (Figure 9-24) is how a set of images will be displayed on the monitor. Users can choose the hanging protocols they prefer for each modality. The hanging protocols can also be required to show the previous examination on one monitor and the current examination on the other. Once the hanging protocols have been set, the most efficient study navigation is determined.

Study Navigation. A **study** in PACS is the current or previous examination being viewed. A study may comprise two or three single images, as is the case with projection radiography, or it may contain several series of images, as is the case with MRI. The images can be paged through either with the scroll wheel or with arrows on the keyboard, or they can be run through in stacks. Many vendors call the stack mode of scrolling through images *cine*. The cine function is used most often in sectional imaging.

Many vendors provide icons (pictures within the software that activate software functions) that allow the user to move among a patient's various studies or open the next unread patient in the worklist after having read the current study. Another navigation tool that is commonly found is a close patient or close study icon. This icon closes the active patient or study and either pulls up the worklist or moves to the next unread patient in the worklist. Users can set up these tools according to their preferences.

Image Manipulation and Enhancement Functions. Once an image has been opened on the display, there are many tools that can be used to change the

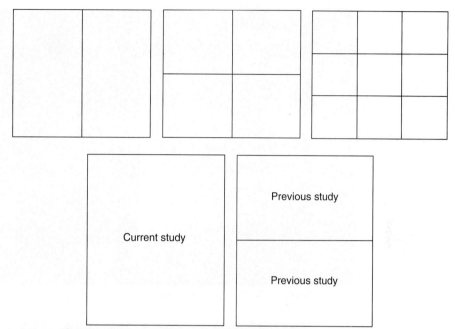

FIGURE 9-24 Typical hanging protocols seen on a PACS workstation.

appearance of the image. Here is a bulleted list of some of the most commonly used functions:

- Window width/window level (Figure 9-25): This is usually a default function of the left mouse button or middle scroll wheel when an image is actively displayed in the software. By depressing and holding down the mouse button and moving the mouse up and down and left and right, the window width and window level can be adjusted. The window width represents the range of gray values that are being viewed, and the window level represents the brightness.

- Annotations (Figure 9-26): Most PACSs can annotate text or graphics onto the image. This function should *not* be used to label left or right to indicate the patient's side; digital R and L will not hold up in court because of the ability to mark anywhere on the image and flip and rotate the image into any layout on the screen. Annotations can indicate prone or supine, 30 minutes, upright or flat, or any other image information the department deems appropriate. Radiologists frequently place arrows or circles around pathology or questionable areas so that the referring physician can pinpoint what is in question.

- Flip and rotate (Figure 9-27): These functions are used to orient the image in the anatomic hanging position desired by the department. There are usually left-to-right flip and 90-degree clockwise and counterclockwise icons. This function makes it very important that lead markers are used to ensure that the radiologist reads the correct side.

- Pan, zoom, and magnify (Figure 9-28): These functions are used primarily by the radiologist to increase the size of an area on the image. The magnify function

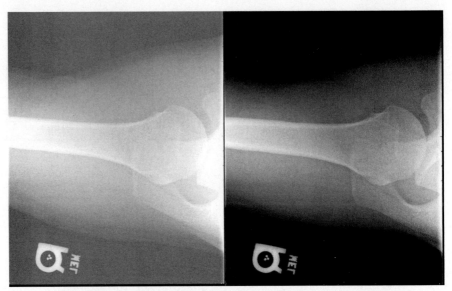

FIGURE 9-25 The same image, but each has a different window/level setting.

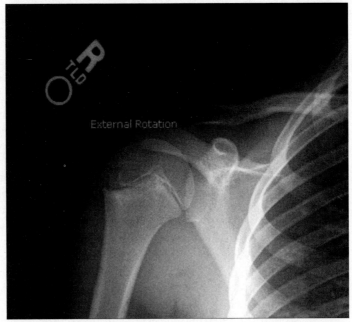

FIGURE 9-26 Text annotations can be placed directly on the image.

will usually enlarge a square area of the image, and the square can be moved around the image to quickly see various areas enlarged. The pan and zoom functions are usually used together. The image is first zoomed up to the desired magnified level, and then the pan icon is activated so that the zoomed image can be moved around, allowing the user to view the different areas of the image.

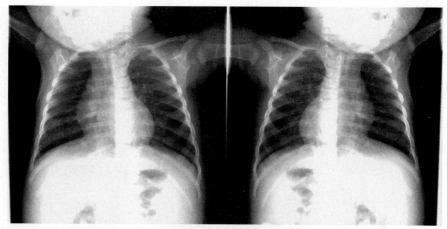

FIGURE 9-27 This image has been flipped left to right.

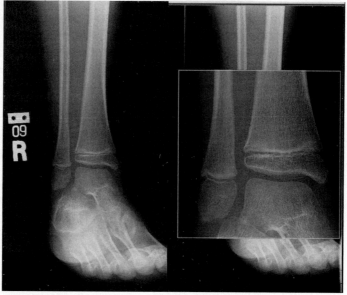

FIGURE 9-28 This section of the image has been magnified to show closer detail of the bone.

- Measurements (Figure 9-29): Various measurement functions are found on a PACS station. The most common is the distance measurement. The size of a pixel is a known measurement, so the software can measure structures on the image based on this known measurement. Another common measurement is the angle measurement, which measures the angle between two structures; this measurement function is commonly used when reading spine studies. Another common measurement a radiologist may use is a region of interest (ROI), which will determine the pixel intensity of a certain area. Because each type of tissue or fluid has a little bit different intensity reading, the radiologist can make a determination whether something is solid or fluid.

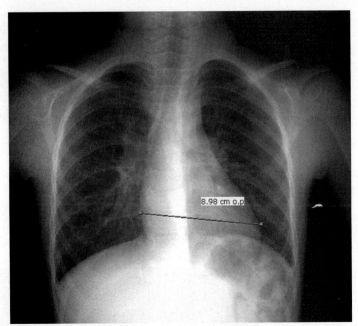

FIGURE 9-29 The distance measurement tool can be used to measure structures on the image.

Image Management Functions. Most PACSs allow the user to modify patient demographics (Figure 9-30) at the technologist QC station, the reading station, and the file room station. It is imperative that the patient demographics are correct. If wrong information is archived on an image, the image will be difficult to retrieve and may never be found again. Make changes only when the information is absolutely known to be wrong. To minimize errors, many hospitals allow only certain people the access to change demographics.

Another image management function is the query/retrieve function used to retrieve studies from the archive (Figure 9-31). The query function allows the user to query a study on multiple fields such as the patient's name or ID, date of service, or modality. Some systems also allow a query based on a diagnosis code or comment field.

Many vendors have provided a CD-burning option that allows users to save studies to a CD for outside use. The feature may be available only in the file room to control the CDs that are sent out. Health Insurance Portability and Accountability Act (HIPAA) compliance must also be maintained. Another common feature is the ability to copy and paste images into a document. This is frequently used with the web-based systems when creating presentations for conferences. The patient information must be removed from the image before it is placed into a presentation.

Some hospitals have retained the ability to print films for outside use. This is also usually done only in the file room so that control can be maintained over the printed films for HIPAA purposes and cost reasons. Some hospitals have also connected workstations to paper printers for quick consults and medical records.

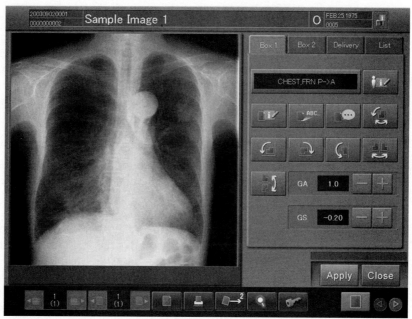

FIGURE 9-30 Patient demographics can be changed after image acquisition on some PACS workstations. *(Courtesy FUJIFILM Medical Systems USA, Inc.)*

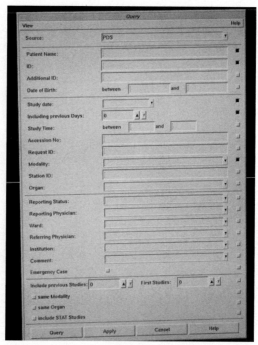

FIGURE 9-31 The user can query images from the archive using various search parameters.

Advanced Workstation Functions

Advanced functions are usually placed on specialty workstations for the radiologist, but some are found on the technologist QC station to further enhance the images. The following are some of the most common advanced functions.

Reading Station Advanced Functions

- Multiplanar reconstruction (MPR) (Figure 9-32): One of the most commonly used three-dimensional (3D) rendering techniques. When doing a CT scan of a patient, thin axial slices can be acquired of a volume of tissue. The slices can then be loaded into the MPR software, and a reconstruction in another plane can be produced. The most common application is producing coronal images from the axial set to reduce radiation to the patient and to reduce scan time at the modality.
- Maximum intensity projection and minimum intensity projection (MIP and MinIp) (Figure 9-33): Used to visualize vessels (MIP) and air-filled structures (MinIp). Commonly performed after the injection of contrast on CT and MRI studies, the contrast will show areas of strictures and blockages within the vessels.
- Volume rendering technique (VRT) (Figure 9-34): Similar to MIP but allows the user to assign colors based on the intensity of the tissue so that bone, contrast agent, and organs can be seen in different colors. The technique uses a histogram-type graph to differentiate the various structures.

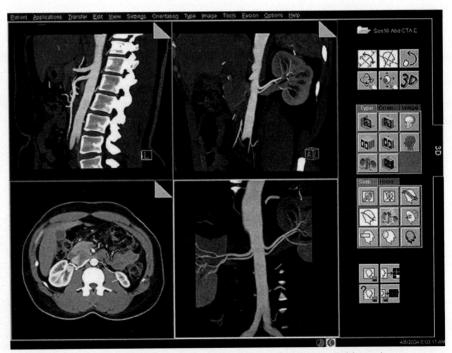

FIGURE 9-32 An MPR image. *(Image courtesy of Siemens Healthcare.)*

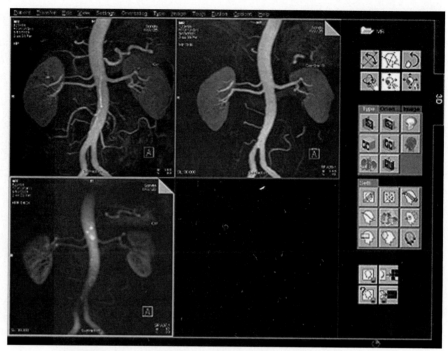

FIGURE 9-33 An MIP image. *(Image courtesy of Siemens Healthcare.)*

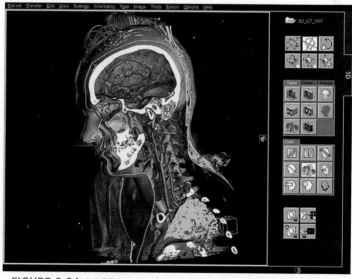

FIGURE 9-34 A VRT image. *(Image courtesy of Siemens Healthcare.)*

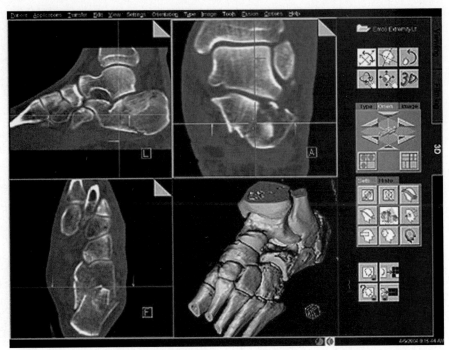

FIGURE 9-35 A 3D shaded surface image. *(Image courtesy of Siemens Healthcare.)*

- Shaded surface display (SSD) (Figure 9-35): Using a threshold of pixel intensity values, everything below the threshold will be removed, and everything above will be assigned a color and shown as a 3D object.

Technologist QC Station Advanced Functions

- Stitching (Figure 9-36): Used when multiple images need to be put together into one image. The most common application is for full-spine x-rays or a scoliosis series. The examination was traditionally performed on a 3-foot film and processed; manufacturers have developed a 3-foot cassette that contains multiple imaging plates (IPs). Each of the IPs is scanned through the reader, and the individual images are sent to the QC workstation. The software then interpolates the images and connects them using known markers from the IPs. The technologist can adjust how the images are connected. Another application of stitching is producing long leg images for leg length discrepancy studies. The images are acquired in a fashion similar to the one described above and stitched together. If the special 3-foot cassettes are not available, a radiopaque ruler must be used to ensure that the images are stitched at the right area.

- Image postprocessing: Is regarded as an advanced function of the workstation, such as edge enhancement, smoothing, and contrast enhancements. These were discussed in earlier chapters.

There are many other advanced workstation functions available to be added to the PACS workstation. This is a growing field with advancements coming each year. Specific information about how to perform these procedures can be found in the vendor's user manual.

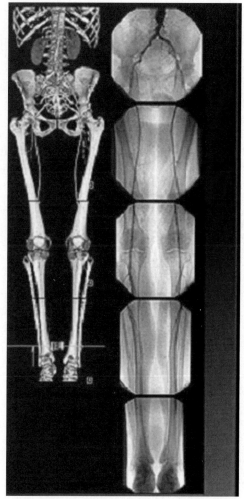

FIGURE 9-36 This image was stitched together from two separate images. *(Image courtesy of Siemens Healthcare.)*

SUMMARY

- A PACS consists of digital acquisition, display workstations, and storage devices interconnected through an intricate network.
- DICOM is a universally accepted standard for exchanging medical images between the modality, viewing stations, and the archive.
- A display workstation is any computer that a health care worker uses to view a digital image, and it is the most interactive part of a PACS.
- The archive is the central part of the PACS and houses all of the historic data along with the current data being generated.
- Workflow is how a process is done step by step or how a task is completed.

- System architecture can be defined as the hardware and software infrastructure of a computerized system.
- Common system architectures found with a PACS are client/server-based systems, distributed or stand-alone systems, and web-based systems.
- Display stations can be categorized by their primary use, such as reading stations for radiologists, review stations for referring physicians, technologist QC station for technologist review of images, and image management station for the file room personnel.
- There are many functions available on a PACS workstation, and each set of functions can be broken down into four categories: navigation functions, image manipulation and enhancement functions, image management functions, and advanced workstation functions.

CHAPTER REVIEW QUESTIONS

1. What does the acronym PACS stand for?
   a. Picture Access Computer System
   b. Permanent Archival Computer System
   c. Picture Archiving and Communication System
   d. Permanent Access Communication System
2. In which type of workstation can changes not be made to the patient demographics of an image set?
   a. Reading workstation
   b. Review workstation
   c. Technologist QC workstation
   d. File room workstation
3. Which PACS device stores the historic image data to be viewed along with current studies?
   a. Display workstation
   b. Archive server
   c. File room workstation
   d. Technologist QC workstation
4. In which PACS architecture is the archive the central repository for all images?
   a. Client/server
   b. Distributed
5. In a web-based system, images are sent directly from the modality to a display workstation for image interpretation.
   a. True
   b. False
6. Monitor type and configuration are of no concern when implementing a PACS in a radiology department.
   a. True
   b. False
7. What workstation function will allow the user the ability to arrange a certain number of images per monitor per modality?
   a. Study navigation
   b. Flip/rotate

    c. Pan

    d. Hanging protocols

8. Digital right and left markers should be used to indicate the anatomic side imaged.

    a. True

    b. False

9. Which advanced image manipulation function will allow the radiologist to view several different anatomic planes from the original acquired sagittal images?

    a. Shaded surface display

    b. Volume rendering technique

    c. Maximum intensity projection

    d. Multiplanar reconstruction

10. Which advanced image manipulation function will allow the technologist to join multiple images together as one?

    a. Stitching

    b. Appending

    c. Volume rendering technique

    d. Multiplanar reconstruction

PACS Archiving and Peripherals

ARCHIVING COMPONENTS

The term **archive** can be defined as a place where records or documents are preserved (Figure 10-1). In a picture archiving and communication system (PACS), the electronic archive serves as the new file room and warehouse for all digital imaging and communications in medicine (DICOM) imaging modalities (Figure 10-2). The PACS archive stores all patient and image data, often on magnetic tape or optical disk. Also, the PACS archive controls the receipt, storage, and distribution of new and historic images. Because of the explosive growth in the use of digital imaging in radiology, the archive is one of the fastest growing components in the PACS. Archive technology continues to make drastic improvements each year; the storage capacity is said to double every 18 to 24 months, and the price per gigabyte also continues to decrease.

The archive is a complex arrangement of computers and storage space. As a whole, it consists of several components, both hardware and software. These can be divided into two major categories: image manager or controller and image storage or archive server. The next two sections discuss image management and image storage. Various types of image storage hardware are described. The chapter ends with a discussion of things to consider when choosing an archiving system.

Image Manager

The **image manager** contains the master database of everything that is in the archive. It controls the receipt, retrieval, and distribution of the images it stores and also controls all the DICOM processes running within the archive.

The image manager generally runs a reliable commercial database such as Sybase (Sybase Inc., Dublin, CA) or Oracle (Oracle Corp., Redwood Shores, CA) with structured query language (SQL). This database contains only the image header information, not the image data. The image data are stored on the archive server, which is discussed in the next section. The database is mirrored, meaning that there are two identical databases running simultaneously so that if one goes down, the

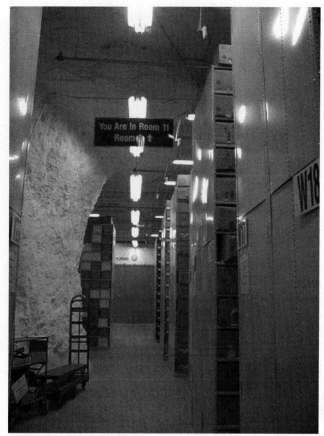

FIGURE 10-1 The archives at the National Archives in Washington, DC.

system can call on the mirror and continue to run as normal, a very important feature.

The image manager is also the PACS component that interfaces with the radiology information system (RIS) and the hospital information system (HIS). This allows the PACS database to collect additional patient information that is necessary for its effective operation. Information extracted from these databases will be used in the prefetching and routing of images to various locations throughout the PACS. The image manager can also play a key role in populating image information into the hospital electronic medical record (EMR).

As mentioned earlier, the image manager database contains the DICOM header information, such as the patient name, identification information (ID), examination date, ordering physician, and location. These fields are organized within the database so that when someone queries for a study on a workstation, the image manager can quickly move through these data fields and locate the images that are being queried (Figure 10-3). The database has pointers associated with each image on the

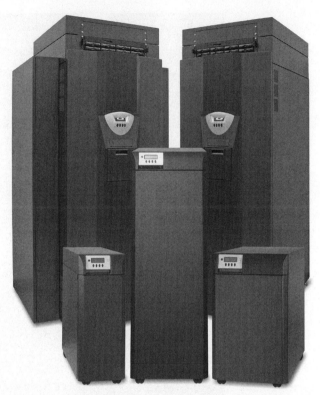

FIGURE 10-2 Examples of PACS archive storage: Magneto-optical disk (MOD) and jukebox. *(Courtesy Sun Microsystems.)*

archive server that point back to the data fields within the database. The following list summarizes the process:

- An order is placed in the RIS for a radiology study.
- The images are acquired and sent to the archive.
- The image manager strips the image header from each image and assigns a pointer to each image or series of images.
- The database files the information in various fields and communicates back to the RIS to verify certain information.
- The study is then queried, and the pointers locate the images on the archive server and send the images to the workstation.

Image Storage

The **image storage** or **archive server** consists of the physical storage device of the archive system. It commonly consists of two or three tiers of storage. A **tier** is a level, layer, or division of something. In an archive server, a tier represents a specific level of archive: short-term, mid-term, or long-term. Most PACS archive systems are set up with a short-term tier and a long-term tier. Short-term means being online or available very quickly, usually within 3 to 5 seconds. Long-term means near line,

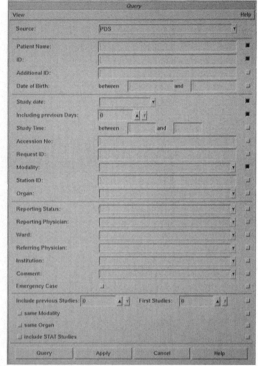

FIGURE 10-3 The PACS database can be queried using various data points.

or images that must be retrieved from a tape or disk storage device and brought to a **redundant array of independent (inexpensive) disks (RAID)**. This could take 1 to 5 minutes.

Short-Term Storage. The short-term tier is commonly a RAID (Figure 10-4). A RAID is composed of several magnetic disks or hard drives that are linked together in an array (Figure 10-5). The size of the RAID ranges from several hundred gigabytes to several terabytes. As the individual disk sizes continue to increase, so does the potential size of the RAID.

In 1988 David Patterson, Garth Gibson, and Randy Katz coined the term RAID in an article entitled "A Case for Redundant Arrays of Inexpensive Disks (RAID)." Their presentation introduced 5 levels of RAID; now there are 11 levels (Figure 10-6), most of which are combinations of the first 5. The following discussion, which includes diagrams and a short synopsis for each of the RAID levels 0, 1, 3, and 5, illustrates how the RAID levels differ from one another:

- RAID 0: Data are "striped" across all of the connected disks. Striping means that the data are broken up into pieces, and each disk will have one piece of the data (Figure 10-7). When the data are called up from the RAID, all of the data are put together from the disks and presented to the user as a whole.
- RAID 1: All of the data sent to the RAID are mirrored onto two disks (Figure 10-8). Mirroring means that all of the data are duplicated and placed onto two separate disks. This RAID level has full redundancy, meaning that if one disk

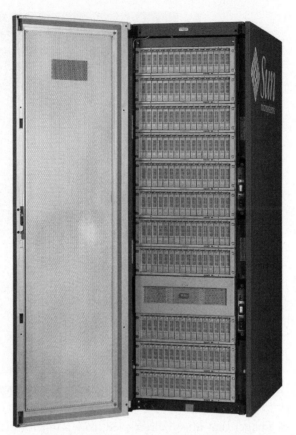

FIGURE 10-4 A redundant array of independent disks (RAID). *(Courtesy Sun Microsystems.)*

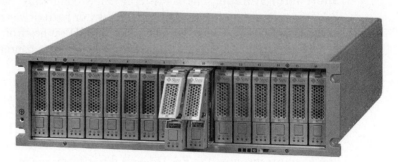

FIGURE 10-5 A RAID array. *(Courtesy Sun Microsystems.)*

goes down, the other one takes over and operation of the system continues. This is a very expensive system because only half of the total storage is used.

- RAID 3: The data are striped across all of the disks just like in RAID 0, but there is one disk that is set aside for error correction. This disk is known as the parity disk (Figure 10-9). This RAID level is rarely used.

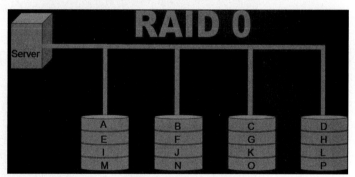

RAID Levels

RAID 0	Striped – no fault tolerance
RAID 1	Mirroring
RAID 2	Error Correcting Coding
RAID 3	Byte level striping & dedicated parity
RAID 4	Block level striping & dedicated parity
RAID 5	Byte level striping & parity
RAID 6	Block-level striping with two parity blocks
RAID 10	Stripe of mirrors
RAID 0+1	Mirror of stripes
RAID 30	Striping of dedicated parity arrays
RAID 100	A stripe of RAID 10s
RAID 7, S, Z, 1.5	Proprietary

FIGURE 10-6 RAID levels.

RAID 0

FIGURE 10-7 RAID 0.

- RAID 5: This RAID level is similar to RAID 3 but instead of having the parity written to one disk, it is striped along all of the disks within the RAID (Figure 10-10). RAID 5 is the most common level used for a PACS archive because it provides adequate redundancy and fault tolerance.

The striping of data increases the reliability and performance of the system. With certain levels of RAID, if one disk fails, the data from that disk can be regenerated using the redundancy of data on the other disks. The error correction detects any transmission errors, and the data will also be regenerated based on the information from the other disks. Striping also enhances performance because if all of the data were on one disk, data added to the disk first would be accessed first, requiring longer wait times for data added to the disk later. Spreading data over several disks allows all data to be accessed at the same time.

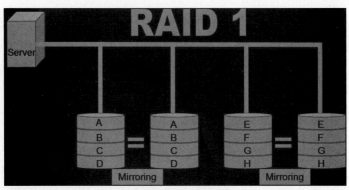

FIGURE 10-8 RAID 1.

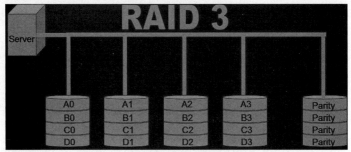

FIGURE 10-9 RAID 3.

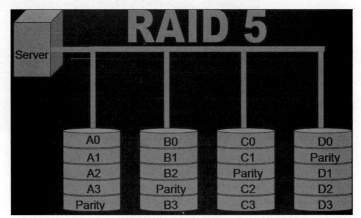

FIGURE 10-10 RAID 5.

Long-Term Storage. Because RAID is becoming more cost-effective, many hospitals use RAID storage for both their short-term and their long-term archive. Other long-term storage products that are still widely used are optical disk, tape, and magnetic disk. Optical disk and magnetic tape archive solutions use a jukebox (Figure 10-11) to hold the tapes or disks; the magnetic disk uses an array. The jukebox has controller software that interfaces with the image manager to keep track of exactly where each image is located. The jukebox controller keeps similar

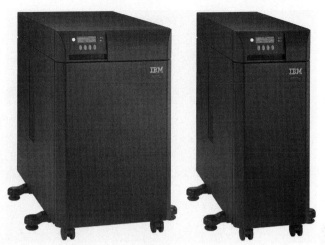

FIGURE 10-11 A DVD jukebox. *(Courtesy of International Business Machines Corporation, © International Business Machine Corporation.)*

studies together as much as possible to minimize access time. The long-term archive has much higher access times than the short-term archive, but the price of storage per gigabyte is much less with the jukeboxes.

Optical Disk

Magneto-optical Disk. A magneto-optical disk (MOD) (Figure 10-12) is very similar to a compact disk (CD) or digital versatile disk (DVD) in that it is read optically with a laser, but the disk itself is housed within a plastic cartridge. MODs tend to be more reliable than some of the other long-term storage options. The disks are rather robust and can withstand many years of reading. They can be read faster than some of their counterparts. The cost per gigabyte is a bit higher for MODs than for some of the other long-term storage options, but MODs are still a viable long-term storage option.

Digital Versatile Disk. Digital versatile disks (DVDs) (Figure 10-13) were first introduced for use in video. CDs were used by a few early PACS adopters, but users found that the CDs could not hold enough data to make a CD archive cost and space efficient. DVDs have a much higher capacity. In 2006, a double-sided, two-layered DVD held 17 GB of data, whereas a CD held 650 MB. DVDs are the least expensive method for long-term archiving per gigabyte.

Ultra Density Optical. Ultra density optical (UDO) disk (Figure 10-14) is the new-generation MOD. A UDO disk uses blue laser technology in its read and write activities. Plasmon (Plasmon PLC, Hertfordshire, UK) introduced the first UDO disk in 2004 with a disk capacity of 30 GB (2006 MOD technology was at 9.1 GB), and the capacity is predicted to increase to 60 GB and then to 120 GB to accommodate industry needs. Currently, UDO technology operating costs are less than MODs and very competitive with DVD technology. The tape libraries being offered in 2006 held between 24 and 638 disks.

Tape. Tape (Figure 10-15) libraries provide the greatest scalability of the long-term archive options. These libraries can grow to hundreds of terabytes, possibly even a petabyte, and this technology will continue to improve and expand its storage limits.

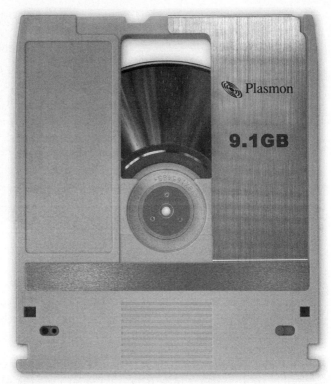

FIGURE 10-12 A magneto-optical disk (MOD). *(Courtesy Plasmon.)*

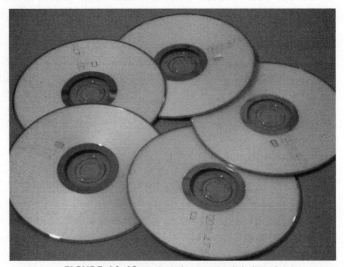

FIGURE 10-13 A digital versatile disk (DVD).

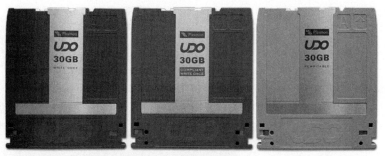

FIGURE 10-14 An ultra density optical (UDO) disk. *(Courtesy Plasmon.)*

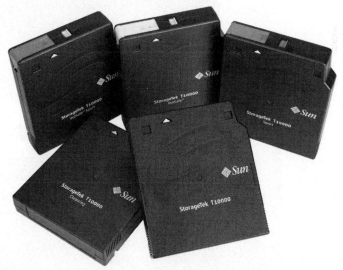

FIGURE 10-15 Magnetic tape. *(Courtesy of Oracle. Oracle, Sun and Java are registered trademarks of Oracle and/or its affiliates.)*

Tape is a fairly low-cost archive medium that comes in various sizes. These tapes are contained within a jukebox or library that has multiple drives and a robot arm to move the tapes in and out of the drives. These libraries can hold between 10 and 1448 tapes in one library (Figure 10-16). Most of the libraries are scalable, meaning that additional libraries can be added to the original.

One of the biggest disadvantages of tape is its unreliability over multiple uses. The tape can wear after several years of heavy use and may become damaged. Tape also has a longer access time than its optical counterparts. Tape has greatly improved in its speed and reliability, and it will continue to be a factor in long-term PACS archiving systems.

There are several types of magnetic tape technologies available:

- Linear tape open (LTO): LTO technology was developed jointly by Hewlett Packard (Palo Alto, CA), IBM (Armonk, NY), and Quantum (San Jose, CA) to make available an open-format tape storage option. Open-format technology means that users have multiple sources of product and media that enable them

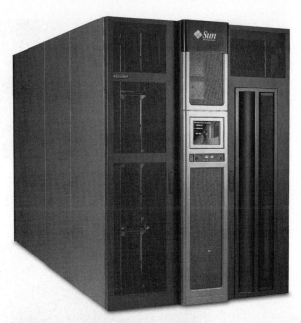

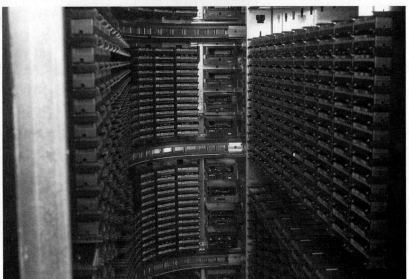

FIGURE 10-16 Various tape libraries. *(Courtesy of Oracle. Oracle, Sun and Java are registered trademarks of Oracle and/or its affiliates.)*

to mix products from various vendors and still maintain compatibility and function. The LTO format is a high-capacity tape technology. Current LTO-3 technology holds 400 GB of uncompressed data on a single tape.

- Digital linear tape (DLT): DLT technology was invented by Digital Equipment Corporation in 1984. It was purchased by Quantum in 1994, and Quantum licenses the technology. DLT tape drives have storage capacities between 40 and

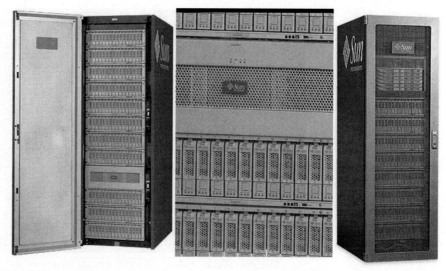

FIGURE 10-17 Magnetic disk storage used as a long-term archive. *(Courtesy of Oracle. Oracle, Sun and Java are registered trademarks of Oracle and/or its affiliates.)*

160 GB, and a newer DLT technology known as super DLT has a capacity of 160 to 300 GB uncompressed.
- Advanced intelligent tape (AIT): AIT is a high-speed and high-capacity tape made by Sony (Tokyo, Japan) to compete with the DLT. Sony introduced AIT in 1996 with a tape capacity of 25 GB; current AIT-4 technology has a capacity of 200 GB. Sony developed the next generation of AIT tapes, known as SAIT, and they have an initial capacity of 500 GB.

Magnetic Disk. As mentioned earlier in the chapter, as the price of **magnetic disk storage** (Figure 10-17) continues to decrease, RAID storage becomes a more feasible option for long-term storage. When using magnetic disks for long-term storage, the RAID arrays may be configured into three different but related fashions: direct attached storage (DAS), network attached storage (NAS), or storage area network (SAN).

- DAS (Figure 10-18): DAS is coupled to the system just like a short-term RAID. The DAS storage is connected directly via cable connections and shows up on the computer as different partitions for use. They are typically managed by the same RAID controller because, in essence, the short-term RAID is just being expanded to have more storage space so that the studies will remain for a longer period of time.
- NAS (Figure 10-19): NAS servers are stand-alone RAID arrays that are attached directly to the network. Multiple NAS servers can be attached to one network to provide additional fault tolerance, and the load can be balanced throughout the servers.
- SAN (Figure 10-20): A SAN is a high-speed, special-purpose network (or sub-network) that links different kinds of data storage devices with associated data

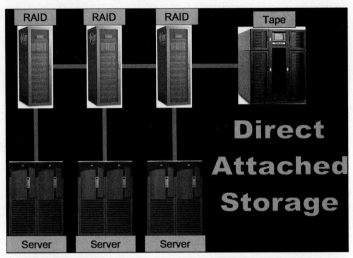

FIGURE 10-18 A direct attached storage long-term archive.

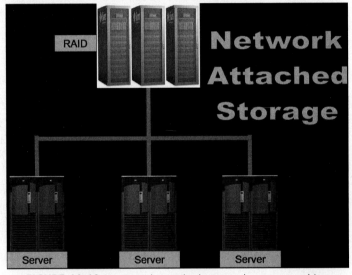

FIGURE 10-19 A network attached storage long-term archive.

servers, such as disk array controllers and tape libraries. SANs are becoming more popular in health care because of plummeting costs of magnetic disk storage. A SAN can be used by multiple departments within an institution and provide exceptional response speed for called-up data. The RAID levels can still be taken advantage of when they are used in conjunction with a SAN.

ARCHIVE CONSIDERATIONS

PACS archives are chosen for many reasons, including system need, system cost, and system compatibility. Many hospitals do not have the capital funds or the

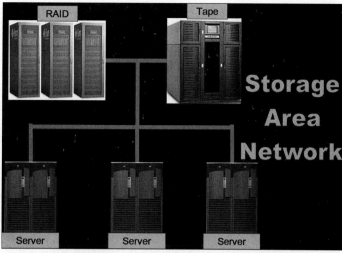

FIGURE 10-20 A storage area network.

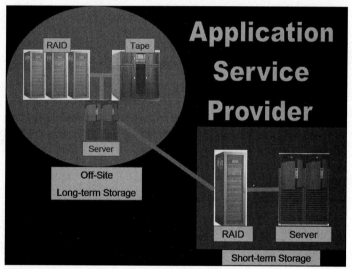

FIGURE 10-21 An application service provider model using off-site, outsourced long-term storage.

personnel to implement and operate the complex archive that is needed for a PACS. These hospitals have sought out other alternatives. One such alternative is an **application service provider (ASP)**. An ASP is a company that provides outsourcing of archiving and management functions for a pay-per-use or pay-per-month charge. ASPs give smaller institutions access to the level of hardware and software they could not otherwise afford. Moreover, they assume responsibility for the day-to-day management of the archive system. Many ASP models have a short-term archive located on hospital premises, and the long-term archive is handled at the off-site location run by the ASP company (Figure 10-21). The short-term archive may be leased by the ASP, and the controller will prefetch images from the long-term off-site storage during the evening and night hours for the next day's schedule.

Another common use for an ASP is as a disaster recovery mechanism. **Disaster recovery** involves making copies of each tape or disk and sending them to another building or off-site location or, by using the ASP model, shipping them to an outside company for storage on a pay-per-use policy. Even larger institutions have difficulty purchasing the proper amount of storage for disaster purposes. With proper disaster recovery, a complete copy of the archive is housed in another location and immediately available if the front-line archive goes down for any reason. With an ASP, however, the data may be housed in another state in a large storage silo, and the duplicated data may not be immediately available. There are many facets to disaster recovery, but a discussion of them is outside the scope of this textbook. The most important thing to know is that backups are completed each day on the image manager database and that there must be some sort of contingency plan should disaster strike the archive room.

The archive is a complex arrangement of servers, databases, and storage devices. It is the most integral part of a PACS and is in general the most difficult piece to fully understand. This chapter presents an overview of the topic but by no means has presented the information needed to successfully purchase or operate a PACS archive.

PACS PERIPHERAL DEVICES

The previous chapters discussed the digital image acquisition process, PACS workstations, and archive systems. This chapter introduces you to three other components that are common in a PACS: film digitizers, imagers, and CD burners. Each of these three technologies plays an important role in the PACS.

FILM DIGITIZERS

Another way to take a projection radiograph to a digital format other than photostimulable phosphor or flat-panel digital technology is by using a film digitizer. The **film digitizer** (Figure 10-22) scans the analog film and produces numeric signals for each part of the scanned film. The numbers are fed into a software application that is attached to the scanner, and the scanner digitally reproduces the image using the numeric signals that represent each part of the radiograph.

There are two major types of film digitizers; one type uses laser technology, and the other type uses charge-coupled device (CCD) technology. Both are equal in quality, but currently the CCD digitizers are less expensive.

Laser Film Digitizers

A laser film digitizer uses a helium neon laser beam to convert the analog film image into a digital image (Figure 10-23). A laser inside the digitizer is bounced off a series of mirrors and scanned across the image. A photomultiplier tube picks up the light that is transmitted through the film. The laser scans one line at a time, and the photomultiplier picks up a very small area and then moves to the next area. The

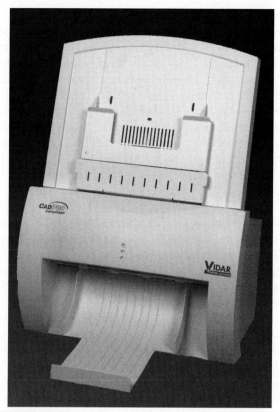

FIGURE 10-22 Typical film digitizer. *(Courtesy 3D Systems.)*

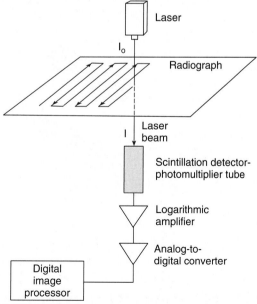

FIGURE 10-23 The process of digitizing a film using a laser film digitizer.

electrical signal is then sent to an analog-to-digital converter where the signal is translated into numbers based on the optical density of the film and the signal received. The numbers are then displayed on a monitor based on a look-up table (LUT) that indicates which shade of gray is associated with each number.

Laser digitizers are considered the gold standard for film digitization, and they have been around since approximately 1990. These digitizers can scan at various resolutions up to 5K and 12 bit, depending on the application need, and can scan an image in less than 25 seconds, depending on the scanning resolution. The disadvantages of laser digitizers include their expense and service needs, including maintenance, calibration, and quality control (QC) tests.

CCD Film Digitizers

A CCD film digitizer uses fluorescent bulbs that shine through the film and a CCD array that detects the light and transforms it into an electrical signal (Figure 10-24). The signal is then sent to an analog-to-digital converter and changed into a number that represents the intensity of light that passed through the film. As with the laser digitizer, the number is referenced against a LUT, and an image is displayed on a monitor.

The CCD digitizers are less expensive than the laser digitizers but somewhat slower. A CCD digitizer can take up to 80 seconds to scan one film through the digitizer, and it can also have problems with extreme light and dark areas on the film. However, the CCD digitizer image quality has improved over the years, and many radiologists say that the quality is adequate for their needs.

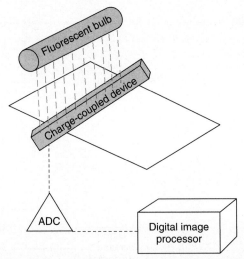

FIGURE 10-24 The process of digitizing a film using a CCD film digitizer. *ADC,* Analog-to-digital converter.

Common Uses of Digitizers

There are many uses for the film digitizer in the modern radiology department. Most departments list the following reasons for using a digitizer:

- Teleradiology: **Teleradiology** is a term used to describe the process of transferring digitized images for delivery at a distance to radiologists. Many hospitals use the digitizer to transfer films from off-site clinics to the main department for primary reading. The films are placed in the digitizer, and the image is transformed into a digital signal and sent via a network back to the main department. This saves the radiologist from having to drive to the remote location to read the few films that have been taken. It is also better patient care because films will be read much more quickly if sent digitally to the radiologist.
- Compare outside or old films: If a hospital has a PACS installed and is reporting the image from a monitor, it is very difficult to compare a film image with the image on the monitor. Many hospitals will digitize the patient's old films so that a comparison can be done much more easily. Patients also frequently come in with outside films. These are routinely digitized into the archive so that they can be referred to at a later date and compared with new digital images.
- Film duplication: On occasion it is necessary to make duplicate copies of films. The film can be sent through the digitizer, and then the image can be printed onto film using a laser film imager.
- Computed aided diagnosis (CAD): A new technology that is gaining momentum is CAD. It is most currently used in mammography and chest imaging. The film is sent through the digitizer, and a computer will analyze the densities seen on the image and alert the radiologist of questionable densities.

IMAGERS

Imagers, also known as film printers, receive an image from a workstation and print the image based on printer LUTs and preset print layouts. Both of these parameters vary for each modality that produces digital images. There are two major types of imagers: wet (chemical) laser imagers (Figure 10-25) and dry laser imagers (Figure 10-26).

Wet Imagers

Wet imagers use chemicals to process the film that has been exposed to the laser. The laser beam produces an intensity of light that is proportional to the signal being received to regulate the optical density recorded on the film. The laser emits a red light, so the film that is used must be red sensitive. As mentioned earlier, conventional film has silver halide crystals suspended in an emulsion; the wet laser film is not much different other than being red sensitive so that the laser may etch the image into the film. Because this film is sensitive to red light, it must be placed in its film magazine and processed in total darkness. This processing takes place in a bath of chemicals just like film used in the traditional film/screen department.

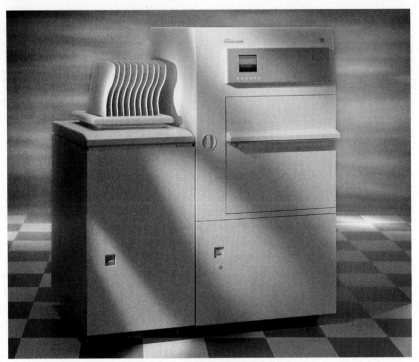

FIGURE 10-25 A wet laser imager. *(Courtesy Carestream Health, Inc.)*

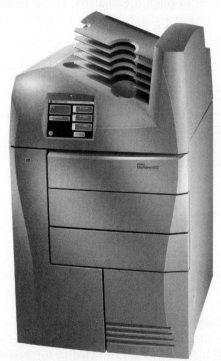

FIGURE 10-26 A dry laser imager. *(Courtesy Carestream Health, Inc.)*

Because wet imagers require chemicals, they must be placed in a well-ventilated area with proper drainage and plumbing. Because of these requirements, fewer departments install this type of imager. Wet imagers also take up much more space than the dry imagers, and the cost of chemicals, disposal, and maintenance make them a less popular choice than dry imagers.

Dry Imagers

Dry imagers use heat to process the latent image that is etched into the silver emulsion by the laser. Just like conventional film, dry laser film also has silver within its emulsion, but instead of silver halide crystals, the dry film has silver behenate. The film is exposed with a laser in a fashion similar to the wet imager. The silver salts are then exposed to heat and turn to metallic silver to create the image on the film.

Dry imagers have been found to have slightly worse quality than wet imagers, but the dry imagers take up less space and require no special locations. The dry imager film quality tends to degrade over time, and it is more sensitive to heat and humidity than conventional film, especially if the film is stored in a warm environment. Moreover, because the silver salts that make the image are still on the film after it is processed, the image can gain more density when stored in a high-heat area. The major advantage to the dry imager is that it only requires an outlet and a network connection to connect to the departmental modalities.

Common Uses of Imagers

Even though the future of radiology is a filmless environment, there will always be a need for producing a hardcopy film. The following list outlines a few reasons why film can and will be used in what nevertheless is called the filmless radiology department.

- Backup: The ability to print just in case the PACS goes down is one of the most often heard explanations. In most hospital networks, the modalities are set up to send not only to the PACS but also directly to a laser imager. Thus if the PACS is down for some reason, the modality can still print directly to the imager.
- Difficult PACS locations: When a PACS is installed, there are a few departments that are difficult to convert to PACS initially, such as surgery, orthopedics, and sometimes the emergency room. In surgery, space is at a premium, and it may be difficult to place a PACS workstation in the surgical suite. In many instances, films are printed for surgery and placed on a lightbox.
- Outside physicians: Many referring physicians prefer to see their patient's images while reviewing the radiologist's report. When installing a PACS, one of the last pieces to be converted is outside physician access so, with imagers, films can be printed and sent to the physicians as normal.
- Legal cases: For legal cases, films can be printed to be viewed in court. It may become more commonplace to have computer access in the courtroom, and at that time images can be viewed digitally.
- Teaching purposes: Most hospitals train students at their institution. The printing of films for training purposes will continue to be a need.

CD/DVD BURNERS

Early PACS advocates used cost savings to justify purchasing a PACS, but we have seen that there remains a need for hard copies. Film printing is a costly part of a PACS because laser film is expensive, more expensive than conventional film. Most hospitals try to reduce the amount of printing done in the department. One alternative to printing hard copies is to burn images to an optical disk.

Remember from Chapter 7 that CDs and DVDs are both thin injection-molded polycarbonate plastic disks. The disk is impressed from a mold to form microscopic bumps that indicate either a 1 or a 0 to the computer. Over the bumps is a reflective layer of aluminum covered with a clear protective coat of acrylic. In a DVD there are multiple layers of the polycarbonate plastic. Aluminum is used behind the inner layers, and gold is used behind the outer layers. The gold is semi-reflective so the laser can penetrate to the inner layers of plastic. With a **burner**, the information is burned onto the disk starting in the center and spiraling out to the edge of the disk. The laser will burn a tiny depression (pit) into the disk to represent the data being saved. A burned disk will be a series of pits and lands, areas that were not burned by the laser (Figure 10-27).

All PACS vendors offer the ability to burn images to a CD or DVD for the purpose of sharing the images outside of the PACS. When a disk is burned with the patient's images, a DICOM viewer is also burned onto the disk. When the disk is put into a drive, the software automatically launches and displays the images. The software is generally very intuitive and easy to use and allows for minor image enhancements such as window/level adjustments and simple measurements.

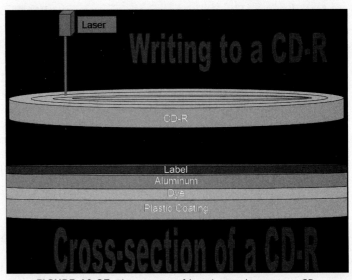

FIGURE 10-27 The process of burning an image to a CD.

Common Uses of Burners

CDs and DVDs can be used in most of the same applications as the printed film with the exceptions that CDs and DVDs cannot be used as a fail-safe mechanism nor can they be used by those departments that are in difficult locations. Many referring physicians prefer having the images on disk rather than film because it takes up less space, can be added directly to the patient's office chart, and the images can be manipulated.

Disks also are much less expensive to produce and send out to physicians. One sheet of dry laser film costs approximately 48 cents, whereas a CD costs approximately 28 cents. The CD can hold multiple studies, and multiple sheets of film would be needed to print an entire study. The CD is also much less expensive to mail than the film. Disks will become much more common outside of the radiology department as the advantages are seen by those outside of the department.

SUMMARY

- The archive is a complex arrangement of computers and storage space that is the permanent location for digital images.
- The image manager contains the master database of everything that is in the archive.
- The archive server consists of the physical storage devices of the archive system.
- Most PACS archives are set up with short-term and long-term archive tiers.
- A short-term tier is commonly a redundant array of independent (inexpensive) disks (RAID).
- A RAID is composed of several magnetic disks or hard drives that are linked together in an array.
- RAID 5 is the most common RAID level used in PACS archives.
- Long-term storage devices hold historic images for comparison reading on the workstations.
- Tape, optical disk, and magnetic disks are commonly used as long-term archive solutions.
- An application service provider (ASP) is a company that provides outsourcing of archiving and management functions for a pay-per-use or pay-per-month charge.
- A proper disaster recovery mechanism keeps a complete copy of the archive in another location that is immediately available in the event that the front-line archive goes down. A film digitizer scans the analog film and produces numeric signals for each part of the scanned film.
- A laser film digitizer uses a helium neon laser beam to convert the analog film image into a digital image.
- A charge-coupled device (CCD) film digitizer uses fluorescent bulbs that shine through the film and a CCD array that detects the light and transforms the light into an electrical signal.
- Imagers, also known as film printers, receive an image from a workstation and print the image based on printer look-up tables (LUTs) and preset print layouts.

- Dry imagers use heat to process the latent image that is etched into the silver emulsion by the laser.
- Wet imagers use chemicals to process the film that has been exposed to the laser.
- A CD/DVD burner can burn images to be shared outside of the radiology department. Along with the images, a DICOM viewer is burned to the disk for ease of viewing.

CHAPTER REVIEW QUESTIONS

1. What part of the archive contains the master database of everything contained within the archive?
   a. Image manager
   b. Image storage
   c. Archive server
   d. Both b and c
2. What part of the archive contains the physical storage of images within the archive?
   a. Image manager
   b. Image storage
   c. Archive server
   d. Both b and c
3. What term is used to describe a layer of archive storage?
   a. Disk
   b. Database
   c. Tier
   d. None of the above
4. The term RAID stands for _____.
   a. redundant area of independent disks
   b. redundant array of illogical disks
   c. redundant array of independent disks
   d. retrievable array of inexpensive disks
5. Which RAID level is often seen in PACS archives?
   a. 0
   b. 1
   c. 3
   d. 5
6. Which of the following are considered long-term storage devices?
   a. MOD
   b. DVD
   c. DLT
   d. RAID
   e. All of the above
7. Which RAID configuration is directly attached to a network?
   a. DAS
   b. NAS
   c. SAN
   d. All of the above

8. Which RAID configuration is a special network of storage devices?
   a. DAS
   b. NAS
   c. SAN
   d. All of the above
9. What device will scan an analog x-ray film into a PACS?
   a. Image server
   b. Image manager
   c. Film imager
   d. Film digitizer
10. What do dry imagers use to process the latent image on the film?
   a. Chemicals
   b. Heat
   c. Laser
   d. Light

PART V

Quality Control and Quality Management

Ensuring Quality in PACSs

On completion of this chapter, you should be able to:

- Describe the differences between quality control (QC) and quality assurance activities.
- Define *continuous quality improvement (CQI)* and its uses in a radiology department.
- Describe the daily and monthly/quarterly QC monitoring activities.
- Discuss the process of daily/weekly QC on laser imagers.
- State the common QC activities used to measure system speed and data integrity.
- Describe several quality assurance (QA) activities used in a digital radiology department.

KEY TERMS

Acceptance testing
Continuous quality improvement
 (CQI)
Error maintenance
PACS administrator
Photometer

Quality assurance (QA)
Quality control (QC)
Routine maintenance
Super user
The Joint Commission (TJC)

QUALITY ASPECTS

When you think of quality, what is the first thing that comes to mind? Is it the service at a restaurant or the backpack purchased at the beginning of the semester? Both examples deal with quality in some way: one is people-centered, and the other is product-centered. Likewise, radiology has both a people-centered quality and a product-centered quality.

The traditional radiology department with film and chemistry has many quality procedures that must be followed. Many of these same protocols are used in the digital department, but they have been modified to be relevant to digital equipment and processes.

The next section introduces the terms used to talk about quality within a radiology department. The following sections introduce various routines that should be followed in the department to ensure that the picture archiving and communication system (PACS) is functioning properly and that the images are being produced at a certain quality level. Chapter 12 discusses quality issues related to digital radiographic equipment and processes.

TERMS OF QUALITY

Quality has always been a part of health care, whether as a service or product. Health care institutions pride themselves on providing the highest quality possible, and they put many measures into place to ensure that the highest quality is provided to each patient. The ultimate focus in health care is to improve patient care and provide a high-quality service so that patients will want to return. Most health care institutions are accredited by **The Joint Commission (TJC)**, formerly known as the Joint Commission on the Accreditation of Healthcare Organizations (JCAHO). This accreditation is voluntary but necessary in many instances to obtain Medicaid certification, hold certain licenses, obtain reimbursements from insurance companies, and receive malpractice insurance. Rather than simply referring to *quality*, today TJC uses the more encompassing terms *continuous quality improvement* or *total quality management*. The next few sections define these concepts and provide examples of some basic applications in a digital department.

Quality Assurance

Quality assurance (QA) can be defined as a plan for the systematic observation and assessment of the different aspects of a project, service, or facility to make certain that standards of quality are being met. QA activities are focused around people and service. In a radiology department there are many processes involved in the day-to-day activities. For example, once a patient has been checked in at the front desk, there is a process that is followed to alert the technologist that a patient is waiting. If this process is not followed, the patient may have to wait for an extended period before a technologist arrives to check for waiting patients. This extended wait time affects patient care in a negative manner, and therefore it will be seen as poor quality of service. A QA measure should be in place to monitor patient wait times to ensure that the process of alerting a technologist that a patient is waiting is working properly.

Most QA activities will produce quantitative data that can be analyzed. These data can be used to monitor the processes and determine whether the process is working as it should and whether the standard of quality has been met.

Quality Control

Quality control (QC) can be defined as a comprehensive set of activities designed to monitor and maintain systems that produce a product. QC measures are instituted to ensure that radiologic procedures are performed safely, are appropriate for the patient, are performed efficiently, and produce a high-quality image. For example, tests are performed on the radiographic room to make sure that all of the parts, such as the collimator, generator, and focal spots, are functioning properly. All of these parts make up the whole of the room, and if one part is off, it can cause harm to the patient or reduce the quality of the examination.

QC measures are required by law to maintain the license for the room or department. The data from the various activities are kept by a designated individual within the department. Most QC activities are part of a QA program, and the data are used to improve the quality of the processes and department. There are three major categories of QC test that are used at various times:

- **Acceptance testing:** This type of testing is performed before newly installed or majorly repaired equipment can be accepted by the department. The testing may be performed by a designated technologist, a radiation physicist, or by service personnel employed by the hospital. The acceptance testing is used to determine whether the equipment is performing within the vendor's specifications and as promised.
- **Routine maintenance:** Routine maintenance is performed to ensure that the equipment is performing as expected. This type of testing can catch problems before they become radiographically apparent. This testing may be performed by a designated technologist, a radiation physicist, or by service personnel employed by the vendor.
- **Error maintenance:** When errors occur in equipment performance, corrective action must occur. Errors will be detected by poor equipment performance or poor quality outcomes. These corrections will generally be made by service personnel employed by the vendor.

Continuous Quality Improvement

Continuous quality improvement (CQI) tends to focus on the process rather than on the people or the service. The belief is that if the process is good, health care workers will follow it, and service will be good. The CQI process does not replace QA/QC programs. The QA/QC programs focus on maintaining a certain level of quality, not necessarily improving to a higher quality. CQI focuses on improving the process or system within which the people function as team members rather than focusing on an individual's work.

One of the most important concepts to understand with CQI is that all levels of people within the organization must be involved in the process of improvement. Because CQI focuses not on individuals and their mistakes but rather on the process, each team member is more apt to participate in improving the organization. It is important that everyone participate because if one spoke is not involved, the wheel will fall off, and the quality cart cannot move forward.

PACS EQUIPMENT QC

When beginning a QC program, care must be taken to document all surrounding variables so that each quality measure can be repeated without harm to the process. Documentation is very important in any QC activity, and all paperwork must be kept up to date to make a valid performance measure. As with all quality activities, documentation is the most difficult part of the process and the easiest part to not complete. Without the documentation to back up the findings, it will be difficult to prove the need for repair or update of a system.

The next several sections focus on QC activities that should be monitored in a PACS environment, including display quality for both monitor and film, processing speed, network transfer speed, and the data integrity of data that are called back from the archive. This is not an all-encompassing list. Many vendors have suggestions for what should be monitored for their systems. It is very important that the vendor's list and timetable for these various activities be followed. According to the American College of Radiology (ACR) Technical Standard for Digital Image Data Management: "Any facility using a digital image data management system must have documented policies and procedures for monitoring and evaluating the effective management, safety, and proper performance of acquisition, digitization, compression, transmission, display, archiving, and retrieval functions of the system. The quality control program should be designed to maximize the quality and accessibility of diagnostic information."

The ACR also suggests that all the quality tests described later in this chapter be carried out with a Society of Motion Pictures and Television Engineers (SMPTE) test pattern (Figure 11-1) to ensure continuity of measurements. A test pattern developed by the American Association of Physicists in Medicine (AAPM) Task Group 18 (TG18) (Figure 11-2) is also becoming more widely accepted for use in these QC tests. The ACR suggests that QC tasks be performed at least monthly, whereas the AAPM has a much more rigorous schedule. The AAPM suggests that the testing be performed on acceptance and annually by a trained physicist, and the

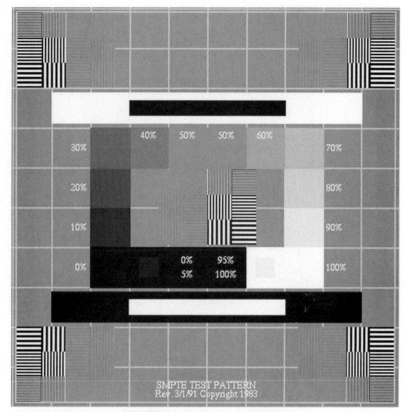

FIGURE 11-1 SMPTE test pattern.

daily and monthly/quarterly tests can be performed by a trained QC technologist or a physicist. If any of the following tests fails or produces out-of-range readings, corrective action and continued monitoring should be done. The technologist should follow the radiology department's policy on equipment maintenance procedures. It may be necessary to contact a radiation physicist to follow up on the findings.

Monitor Quality

The monitor is often the weakest link in the digital imaging chain. The monitor has a direct effect on the quality of the image that is presented to the radiologist for reading or to the referring physician for review. Unfortunately, it is not cost-effective to provide the highest quality monitor for all viewing situations. As discussed in Chapter 2, the radiologist workstation will have the highest quality medical grade monitors, usually 2K or 3K for digital projection images, 1K or 2K for cross-sectional images, and up to 4K for mammography. As with digital cameras, the megapixel measurement may also be used to determine the appropriate monitor. Generally, the physician review workstations and the technologist QC workstations have high-quality commercial monitors; these usually have a resolution of 1K.

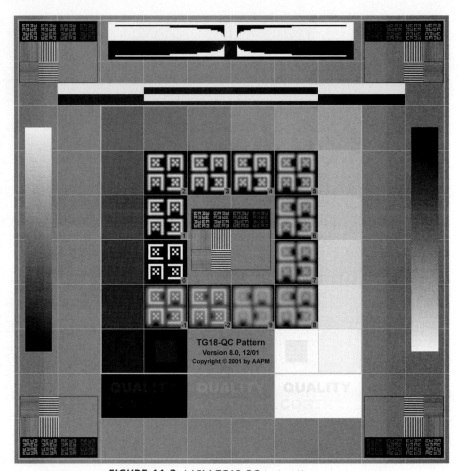

FIGURE 11-2 AAPM TG18-QC test pattern.

The following QC recommendations for display monitors come from the AAPM in its document titled "Assessment for Display Performance for Medical Imaging Systems." This document outlines testing to be completed both by physicists and by technologists/users. The following sections outline the tasks to be completed by a trained technologist on a daily and monthly/quarterly basis on all monitors used to view images; annual and acceptance testing is conducted by a medical physicist.

Daily Monitor QC

- Turn on the monitor, and allow it ample time to warm up.
- Make sure that the monitor is dust-free on the viewing surface and near the airflow areas.
- Retrieve a QC monitor test pattern (SMPTE or AAPM TG18-QC). (The retrieval time may also be noted for a later test to be discussed.)
- General image quality and appearance: Evaluate the overall appearance of the pattern, and take note of any nonuniformities or artifacts, especially at

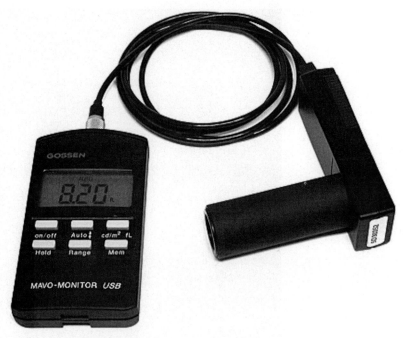

FIGURE 11-3 A photometer used to measure luminescence.

black-to-white and white-to-black transitions. Verify that the vertical and horizontal bars appear continuous.
- Geometric distortion: Make sure that the borders and lines of the pattern are clear and straight and that the pattern appears to be centered in the active area of the display.
- Luminance, reflection, noise, and glare: Verify that all 16 luminance patches are clearly visible. If desired, measure their luminance using a luminance meter or **photometer**, a device used to measure the luminescence of areas on the monitor (Figure 11-3). Evaluate the results in comparison to previous measurements. Make sure that the 5% and 95% patches are clearly visible, and evaluate the appearance of low-contrast letters and the targets at the corners of all luminance patches with and without ambient lighting.
- Resolution: Evaluate the cross patterns at the center and corners of the pattern, and verify that all letters and numbers appear.

Monthly/Quarterly Monitor QC
- Turn on the monitor, and allow it ample time to warm up.
- Make sure that the monitor is dust-free on the viewing surface and near the airflow areas.
- Retrieve a QC monitor test pattern.
- Geometric distortions: Using the TG18-QC test pattern, maximize it to fill the entire usable display area. For rectangular display areas, the patterns should cover at least the narrower aspect of the display area and be placed at the center of the area used for image viewing. The pattern should be examined from a normal viewing distance, and the linearity of the pattern should be checked

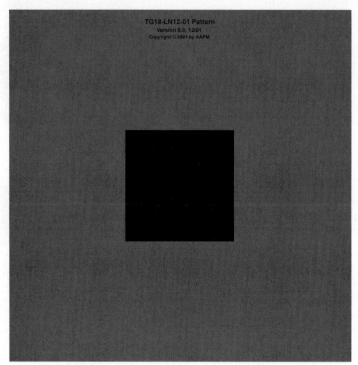

FIGURE 11-4 AAPM TG18-LN-01 test pattern.

visually across the display area and at the edges.

- Reflection: Determine whether there are other light sources such as overhead lights, other monitors, or viewboxes that are reflecting back off of the monitor. Eliminate or reduce these sources of light if possible, and view the test pattern at a normal viewing distance.
- Luminance response: Using the TG18-LN test patterns (Figures 11-4 to 11-6) and a photometer, measure the luminescence from the center of the monitor for each pattern, and record each reading. Also take a reading using the photometer with the monitor in power-save mode or turned off. This will give a baseline reading for the ambient luminance coming from the monitor. A cathode ray tube (CRT) monitor should have a luminance reading of greater than 170 cd/m^2, and a liquid crystal display (LCD) should have a luminance reading of greater than 100 cd/m^2. There should also be a greater than 250 cd/m^2 difference between TG18-LN-01 and TG18-LN-18 test pattern readings (contrast ratio). Using the TG18-CT (Figure 11-7) pattern, the half-moon targets in the center and the four low-contrast objects at the corners of each of the 16 different luminance regions should be visible. Also the bit-depth resolution of the display should be assessed using the TG18-MP (Figure 11-8) test pattern. The assessment includes determining whether the horizontal contouring bands, their relative locations, and grayscale reversals are within limits. Both patterns should be examined from a normal viewing distance.

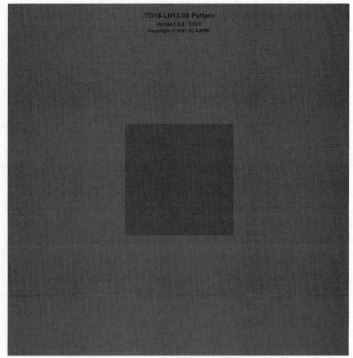

FIGURE 11-5 AAPM TG18-LN-08 test pattern.

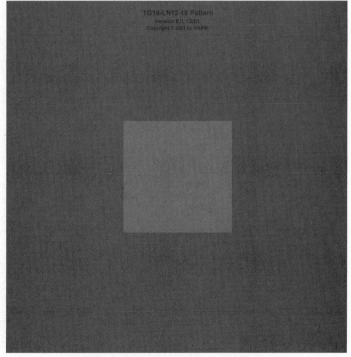

FIGURE 11-6 AAPM TG18-LN-18 test pattern.

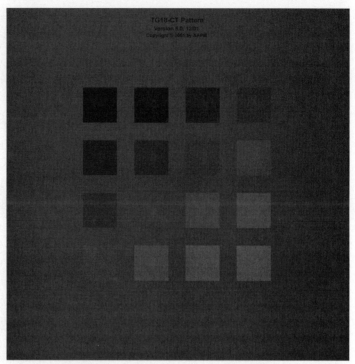

FIGURE 11-7 AAPM TG18-CT test pattern.

FIGURE 11-8 AAPM TG18-MP test pattern.

- Luminance dependencies: Nonuniformity—the visual method for determining display luminance uniformity—uses the TG18-UN10 and TG18-UN80 test patterns (Figure 11-9). The patterns are displayed, and the uniformity across the displayed pattern is assessed. The patterns should be observed from a normal viewing distance. Angular response may be assessed visually using the TG18-CT test pattern. The pattern should first be viewed on-axis to determine the visibility of all half-moon targets. The viewing angle at which any of the contrast thresholds become invisible should be noted. With the TG18-UNL10 and TG18-UNL80 test patterns (Figure 11-10), luminance is measured at five positions over the monitor (center and four corners) using a calibrated photometer. The five readings should be within 30% of one another.

- Resolution: Using the TG18-QC pattern and the magnifying glass within the PACS software, examine the displayed Cx patterns at the center and four corners of the monitor. The line pair patterns in the horizontal and vertical directions should also be evaluated in terms of visibility, and the average brightness of the patterns should also be assessed using the grayscale step pattern as a reference. Note any difference in appearance of the test patterns between the horizontal and vertical lines. The relative width of the black and white lines in these patches should also be examined using the magnifying glass. The resolution uniformity may be determined by using the TG18-CX (Figure 11-11) test pattern and

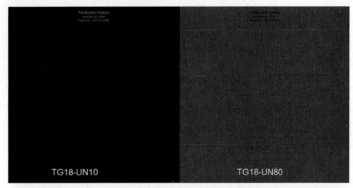

FIGURE 11-9 AAPM TG18-UN10 and TG18-UN80 test patterns.

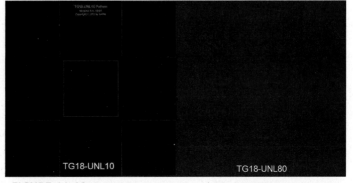

FIGURE 11-10 AAPM TG18-UNL10 and TG18-UNL80 test patterns.

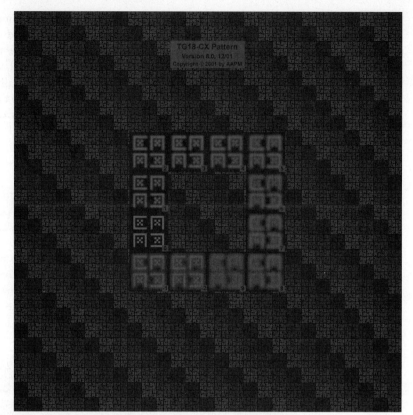

FIGURE 11-11 AAPM TG18-CX test pattern.

magnifying glass in the same way that the Cx elements in the TG18-QC pattern were used.

As mentioned earlier, all annual testing and acceptance testing should be performed by a qualified medical physicist. They follow their own standard set of tests to make sure that the monitors are performing up to their capabilities.

Printer Image Quality

Besides the PACS, the printed image is another way to distribute images around the hospital enterprise. As with monitors, there are several steps that should be taken to ensure that the image being seen is of consistent quality.

Wet Laser Imager

Daily/Weekly QC

- Monitor each film printed to ensure that it is free from artifacts and that it matches monitor or desired quality.
- Print a test pattern from the PACS. Some printers have a built-in test pattern that can be printed by depressing a button on the printer.
- Observe the printed test pattern for artifacts and changes in density, contrast, and resolution.

- Measure the steps on the test pattern using a densitometer, and document your findings. Create a characteristic curve to compare previous measurements.
- Monitor the processing mechanism as you would any chemical processor. Note the temperature, as well as the fixer, developer, and wash levels. Clean the racks and rollers as appropriate.
- Make sure that the preventative maintenance schedule is completed in a timely manner, and maintain documentation of the completion and findings.

Dry Laser Imager
Daily/Weekly QC
- Monitor each film printed to ensure that it is free from artifacts and that it matches monitor or desired quality.
- Print a test pattern from the PACS. Some printers have a built-in test pattern that can be printed by depressing a button on the printer.
- Observe the printed test pattern for artifacts and changes in density, contrast, and resolution.
- Measure the steps on the test pattern using a densitometer, and document your findings. Create a characteristic curve to compare previous measurements.
- Make sure that the preventative maintenance schedule is completed in a timely manner, and maintain documentation of the completion and findings.

Speed

Speed is always a concern in the radiology department, whether it is the speed at which patients are brought back for their x-rays or the speed at which the radiologist gets a final report signed. It is no different in a digital department, but there are other considerations when talking about speed: the processing speed of the workstation and the image retrieval/transfer rate.

Workstation Processing Speed. The workstation processing speed can be measured or documented in many different ways. The following is a practical way for a technologist to monitor the speed of his or her workstation:

- Determine a study to be used as the test. The same study must be used each time to ensure there are no variables. Choose a study with several images and a patient that has several studies.
- Open the initial test study, and note the loading speed. Page through the images, and note the loading speed of each image.
- Choose an image processing function appropriate for the test images that you have chosen, such as edge enhancement, stitching, or a three-dimensional (3D) processing function. Perform the function, and note the processing speed. To maintain consistency, use the same tool each time the test is performed.
- Open the patient's next study using the appropriate PACS function. Note the loading speed of the images.

After acceptance of the workstation, this procedure should be followed weekly to establish a pattern. If no changes are seen, this procedure can then be done on a monthly basis. Any time the software or equipment is updated, the procedure should be done on a weekly basis until a pattern is established again.

Image Transfer Speed. Image transfer speed should be monitored from the modality to PACS and from the archive to a workstation. The following steps are an easy way to monitor these transfer speeds:

- Determine a study to be used as the test. The same study should be used each time to ensure there are no variables. The technologist can also use test patterns that have been saved on the archive. The procedure should be done on the same day of the week and at approximately the same time to reduce network traffic variables.
- Retrieve the study from the workstation. Note the amount of time it took the entire study to arrive at the workstation.
- To test the transfer speed from the modalities, have each modality send its QC images to the archive, and note the amount of time the transfer takes. Make sure that the modality sends the exact same image set each time the test is conducted.

After acceptance of the system, this procedure should be followed weekly to establish a pattern. If no changes are seen, this procedure can then be done on a monthly basis. Any time the software or equipment is updated, the procedure should be done on a weekly basis until a pattern is established again.

Data QC

Data Integrity. A constant measure to be monitored is whether all images completed at the modality make it to the PACS. This is usually caught by the radiologist, but it is a good practice to have the technologist monitor this factor periodically. After initial installation, the technologist should check on a daily basis to make sure that all of the images that he or she sent to the PACS arrived on the PACS. If there are no missing images for several weeks, this practice can be scaled back to once a week. The technologist can randomly choose several studies that were sent during the week to determine whether all of the images made it to the PACS.

Another test for data integrity is to periodically pull up images from the archive to make sure the same images sent initially are still in the study after archival. This should also be done on a weekly basis.

After acceptance of the system, this procedure should be followed daily to establish a pattern. If no changes are seen, this procedure can then be done weekly and then on a monthly basis. Any time the software or equipment is updated, the procedure should be done on a daily basis until a pattern is established again.

Compression Recall. Compression is used to reduce the size of the image files to increase the speed of the network transfer of the images. Compression protocols need to be established by the radiologists and radiation physicist. They will determine the level of compression that will be acceptable for the institution. The following steps are a practical way of observing compression recall of images:

- Save several versions of the AAPM TG18-QC test pattern on the archive using different compression ratios as follows:
  - No compression
  - Lossless compression (2 : 1 compression ratio)

- Lossy compression (variable compression ratios—use the ratio that the department uses, if any)
- Recall all test patterns, and compare the results of no compression, lossless, and lossy. Determine whether there is any loss of information on the compressed images. Note any changes in image quality, if any.

PACS CQI

There are many processes used each day in a PACS environment, and each of these processes should be monitored to make sure that the PACS is functioning up to its capabilities. Remember that CQI activities revolve around process rather than people and systems. The next few sections describe several simple CQI activities that need to be monitored in a radiology department. Many activities that are monitored before the digital conversion of the department should continue after the conversion. Different PACS vendors may have different activities that they recommend. All of these activities should be adhered to so that the PACS will run up to its potential, and problems can be found before they cause major system downtime.

Recognition of Nondiagnostic Images

One CQI activity that should be monitored is the documentation of nondiagnostic images being forwarded to the PACS. This activity will be primarily carried out by the radiologists. If a poor-quality image is detected by the radiologist, the study and performing technologist are noted, and the information is shared with the lead technologist or the PACS administrator to follow up with the performing technologist.

The radiologist may note the areas and reasons for the poor-quality image. If the poor-quality image was caused by equipment malfunction, the appropriate QC test should be carried out, and the appropriate service protocol followed. If the poor-quality image was operator error, additional training or counseling by the supervisor may be required.

System Up-Time

Another common QA activity is the monitoring of how often the system is down for any reason. A log should be kept to note any time that the system is down. Also in the log note the reason, how long, what had to be done to fix the problem, and who fixed the problem. If the same problem continues to occur, this log can be used to prove either that a piece of equipment needs to be replaced or that additional service is needed.

System Training

System training is an important activity that must never stop. One of the early misconceptions related to installation of a PACS is that the vendor applications training will be sufficient for training all staff that interact with the PACS. This is far from the truth. The vendor applications personnel are usually on site for 1 to 2 weeks during initial installation. The vendor applications training is supposed to train several **super users** (people who are trained on all aspects of the system and are prepared to train others) and help set up the system to site specifications.

The super users and the **PACS administrator** (the person trained to oversee the PACS) need to set up an ongoing training program. The training program must include several skill levels, from the radiologist to the technologist to the ancillary personnel. Each new employee needs to be trained on the system. Each time that a new version of the software is installed, the training protocol needs to be revised; retraining of existing personnel may be necessary. Each department also has a list of skills that are tested and retrained each year. PACS skills should be included in this annual training. A training record should be kept for each employee to show proof of skills.

SUMMARY

- Most hospitals are voluntarily accredited by The Joint Commission (TJC). This accreditation is necessary to obtain Medicaid certification, hold certain licenses, obtain reimbursements from insurance companies, and receive malpractice insurance.
- Quality assurance (QA) can be defined as a plan for the systematic observation and assessment of the different aspects of a project, service, or facility to make certain that standards of quality are being met.
- Quality control (QC) can be defined as a comprehensive set of activities designed to monitor and maintain systems that produce a product.
- Acceptance testing is performed before newly installed or substantially repaired equipment is accepted by the department.
- Routine maintenance is performed to ensure that the equipment is performing as expected.
- Error maintenance occurs when errors are detected in equipment performance.
- Continuous quality improvement (CQI) tends to focus on the process rather than the people or the service. CQI focuses on improving the process or system in which people function as members of a team rather than focusing on the individual's work.
- The following QC activities should take place on a prescribed basis:
  - Daily and monthly/quarterly monitor QC
  - Printer image quality
  - Speed assessment
  - Data QC
- Most CQI activities that were in place before the conversion to a digital department should continue. Others should be developed, such as system up-time and system training.

CHAPTER REVIEW QUESTIONS

1. What organization accredits most hospitals in the United States?
   a. CQI
   b. TJC
   c. TQM
   d. OSHA

2. A systematic observation and assessment of different aspects of a radiology department would be what kind of activity?
   a. Quality assurance
   b. Quality control
   c. Quality adjustment
   d. Quality enhancement

3. A comprehensive set of activities designed to monitor and maintain systems that produce a product would be what kind of activity?
   a. Quality assurance
   b. Quality control
   c. Quality adjustment
   d. Quality enhancement

4. What is done after the installation of new equipment to determine if the equipment is performing to vendor specifications?
   a. Error maintenance
   b. Routine maintenance
   c. Acceptance testing
   d. All of the above

5. Continuous quality improvement tends to focus on the people or the service rather than on the process.
   a. True
   b. False

6. What device is used to measure the luminance of a monitor?
   a. Ammeter
   b. Voltmeter
   c. Photometer
   d. Barometer

7. What can be used to determine if the monitor is displaying any distortion over the display?
   a. Photometer
   b. QA procedure
   c. SMPTE pattern
   d. All of the above

8. Printer image quality is of no importance in a digital environment.
   a. True
   b. False

9. Which of the following is a quality control activity performed in a PACS environment?
   a. Image transfer speed
   b. Image processing speed

    c. Data integrity measure

    d. All of the above

10. What PACS CQI activity documents images that are of poor quality?

    a. System training

    b. System up-time

    c. Recognition of nondiagnostic images

    d. All of the above

Quality Acceptance Testing within Digital Projection Imaging

OBJECTIVES

On completion of this chapter, you should be able to:
- Discuss total quality management and its uses in digital projection imaging.
- Describe the daily, weekly, and monthly quality control (QC) activities assigned to a radiologic technologist.
- Explain the importance of establishing a repeat analysis database with digital projection imaging.
- State the common QC activities performed by a service engineer on digital projection imaging equipment.
- Become familiar with problem reporting responsibilities.
- Recognize the quality management (QM) and QC activities to be performed by the radiation physicist.
- Acknowledge personal responsibilities for correctly marking images, maintaining personal repeat rates, and artifact prevention.

KEY TERMS

Total quality management (TQM)   Preventative maintenance (PM)

TOTAL QUALITY MANAGEMENT

Maintenance of equipment, image acquisition, and processing standards are quality control issues that fit into the concept of **total quality management (TQM)** or continuous quality improvement (CQI), as discussed in Chapter 11. The overall efficiency and effectiveness of imaging systems are evaluated beyond the mechanics of producing radiographic images. This chapter introduces the concept of whole system evaluation, considering image acquisition, processing, and evaluation issues as well as examination repeat analysis, communication issues, and system problem identification.

QUALITY CONTROL STANDARDS

The American College of Radiology requires compliance with standards of practice to assure quality in any imaging system. Three general areas define digital image quality: contrast, resolution, and noise. These areas must be monitored to avoid unnecessary repeat examinations and overexposure to patients and staff. There are a number of system tests that must be performed by service personnel and/or radiologic technologists and radiation physicists. With the increased sophistication of digital radiographic equipment, it is critical that these tests be performed in a consistent and thorough manner.

The American Association of Physicists in Medicine publishes the following documents based on work accomplished by task groups:

- Task Group 116—An Exposure Indicator for Digital Radiography
- Task Group 150—Acceptance Testing and Quality Control of Digital Imaging Units
- Task Group 10—Acceptance Testing and Quality Control of Photostimulable Storage Phosphor Imaging Systems

The following sections are in no way an exhaustive list of activities that should be performed. The manufacturer's suggested list of systems tests should be performed as indicated in the equipment and service manuals.

QUALITY CONTROL SCHEDULES AND RESPONSIBILITIES

The radiologic technologist is the first line of defense in preventing, recognizing, and reporting quality control (QC) issues. Quality control is defined as a comprehensive set of activities designed to monitor and maintain a system or piece of equipment. The complicated and delicate nature of digital equipment necessitates frequent and consistent oversight to avoid image errors and unnecessary patient exposure. The following is a suggested schedule for proper digital system maintenance.

BOX 12-1	Summary of Radiologic Technologist Daily QC Duties

Inspect and clean cassettes
Inspect hinge and latch
Erase imaging plates
Verify digital interfaces and network transmission
Inspect laser printer

Technologist Responsibilities

Daily (Box 12-1)

- General system inspection including the following:
  - Sensitometry
  - Laser-generated sensitometry strip; film densities measurement
  - Inspect images
  - Dust particles, scratches, mechanical friction marks
  - Network queue check
  - Send images to picture archiving and communication system (PACS)
  - Cleanliness of cassettes
    - Are the cassettes free of dirt and debris on all surfaces? Dirt on the outside or inside of the cassette can result in an artifact in the image. The artifact could be an exposure artifact or processing artifact depending on when it occurs.
    - Are barcode labels in good condition and able to be read? Labels in disrepair will compromise the connection of the imaging plate identification to the patient and exam identification information.
  - Hinge and latch inspection
  - Are hinges and/or latches in good condition? Broken latches or hinges can damage readers and will require a service call to get the reader in working order.
  - Erasure of imaging plates
  - Have plates been left unexposed for longer than 24 hours? The imaging plates that have not been erased recently have the potential to record exposure such as prolonged light exposure or scatter radiation. The safest procedure is to erase cassettes before use if unsure of the last erasure performed.
  - Verification of digital interfaces and network transmission
  - Is the reader communicating with the workstation? Are barcode readers working properly? Again, it is critical to maintain the link between the imaging plate and patient information.
  - Inspect the laser printer for ink and paper. Make sure the printer is clean and the output bin is free of obstructions. If the printer can be used manually for copies, inspect the printer glass for dirt, fingerprints, etc., and clean according to the manufacturer's specifications. Artifacts produced by dirt and fingerprints can appear and be interpreted as pathology, possibly resulting in false positive diagnoses.

<table>
<tr><td colspan="2">**BOX 12-2**   **Summary of Radiologic Technologist Weekly QC Duties**</td></tr>
</table>

Clean and inspect receptors
Clean air intakes of imaging plate reader
Clean display screen
Clean computer keyboard and mouse

Weekly (Box 12-2)
- Clean and inspect receptors
  - Clean cassettes as needed and inspect the image receptors for dirt or damage. Inspect the entire length of the connection cables for splits or exposure of wires. If breaks or wear have caused wire exposure, inform service personnel immediately. In addition to the danger of electrical shock to personnel, electrical shorts can cause failure of equipment and/or noise on the image.
- Equipment manufacturers should provide lists of appropriate system tests to be performed by the technologists. This type of testing may be performed by a designated QC technologist rather than by each individual technologist. All problems must be recorded and reported immediately. Examples of this type of test include the following:
  - Image acquisition testing with phantoms
  - Cassette integrity testing with special, standardized cassettes
- Clean the air intakes on the image plate reader.
  - Air is used to cool the reader electronics. If dirt and debris are allowed to clog the intakes, the reader could sustain serious damage. In addition, debris entering the air intake could obscure the lens of the scanning laser or reader mirrors and produce artifacts.
- Clean the display screen, keyboard, and mouse.
  - With multiple people using digital imaging systems, and because the digital imaging system makes use of touch screen technology, display screens get dirty very quickly. Multiple users leave multiple fingerprints that, because of the oil in the skin, attract and retain dust and dirt particles. From a visual standpoint, it is much easier to view images on a screen not obscured by streaks and smears. From a health standpoint, many hands on the same surfaces without proper cleaning can lead to increased transmission of illness. Care must be taken to properly clean and disinfect these surfaces according to manufacturers' guidelines.

Monthly (Box 12-3)
- Reject analysis
  - It is critical that repeat exposures are identified so that data concerning repeat reason, number of repeats, and the technologist responsible for the repeat can be analyzed. One issue is that whereas digital systems with integrated generator consoles record the milliampere-seconds (mAs) and kilovoltage peak (kVp) values directly on the film, nonintegrated systems do not. In cases

BOX 12-3	**Summary of Radiologic Technologist Monthly QC Duties**

Reject analysis
Reject reasons
Positioning errors
Marker errors
Equipment malfunction errors
Clean imaging plates
Artifact identification
Problem reporting

Repeat Exam Log

Technologist: _____ Date: _____ Room # _____ Portable _____

Patient ID	Exam	Positioning	Overexposed	Underexposed	Reprinted	Motion	Wrong exam code	Over collimated	Artifact	No exposure	Double exposed	No marker	Marker over part	Other

FIGURE 12-1 Sample repeat rate log.

where the department does not require manual technologist identification input, it is strongly recommended that a personal repeat rate log be kept by each technologist (see sample in Figure 12-1). This will allow the technologist to see possible trends in exposure, positioning, and procedural errors. For example, if the repeat reason is underexposure, the cause could be poor calibration of the automatic exposure control (AEC), or it could be poor imaging skills. Either way, identification of this trend will allow the technologist to improve imaging procedures and better protect the patient. This can be accomplished to a certain extent with a software program. Many vendors have software to automatically keep repeats in a folder for the QC technologists to review, eliminating the issue of technologists deleting repeat exposure images.

QC suboptimal images

Typically, a technologist is assigned the responsibility of coordinating analysis of images of suboptimal quality. This may be done in concert with a radiation physicist, the purpose being to identify equipment and technologist performance errors (see sample reject analysis form in Figure 12-2). This type of analysis helps determine the following:

Reject reasons

Reject reasons are fairly easy to identify in images that demonstrate the mAs and kVp values in the image and digital imaging and communications in medicine (DICOM) header. In images not displaying the technical factors, images that are out of the recommended exposure range can be identified, but unless the technical factors are manually input, there is no way to tell if the problem was caused by mAs or kVp errors. Without the use of side/position markers, there is no way to positively link an image with the performing technologist.

Positioning errors should be easy to identify. Again, without input as to performing technologist, it will be difficult to identify skills issues. It is strongly recommended that the department put a procedure in place that accomplishes this, not for punitive purposes, but for standardization of exposure practices. A major part of being a professional in the imaging sciences is having the integrity to accept responsibility for one's own work. Positioning errors may also be the cause of incorrect processing, related to the position of the part on the imaging plate, collimation, or alignment resulting in poor images even if technique is correct. Vendors are developing software to minimize this, but software is no substitute for proper positioning, collimation, and alignment.

Anatomic side/position marker errors may be very difficult to identify. Because postexposure marking is easily done, technologists may not see the benefit of using personal ID markers. However, this may lead to serious, difficult-to-identify errors. In one case, a technologist performed a portable chest x-ray examination on an infant. Upon processing, she noticed that her personal marker was on the wrong side of the chest. Upon investigation, she discovered that she had marked the chest correctly, but the infant had dexrocardia that had never been identified during six previous exams in which the technologists had failed to use their personal ID markers. There is no substitute for using proper personal ID markers correctly. Incorrect or lack of use of side identification markers may result in legal issues if images are included in a court case. With no blocker for the technologist to use as an identifier of cassette and image orientation, there would be no way to prove proper marking without the technologist ID markers.

Clean imaging plates

Image plates should be removed from the cassette and inspected visually for dirt, hair, lint, scratches, or cracks. Weekly inspection is recommended, especially for departments with high throughput or frequent "dirty" case use. It is important that lint-free cotton gloves be worn to avoid further contaminating the imaging plate. A lint-free cloth such as a photographic lens cloth should

CR/DR Image Analysis Form

Exam/view _____ cm _____ kVp _____ mAs _____

Patient hx _____ Film _____ CR _____ DR _____

Room or reader _____ Date _____ Technologist _____

	Area to evaluate	Criteria	Pass	Reject
1.	**Image identification**			
		Institution name		
		Patient name or number		
		Date		
2.	**Radiographic markers and placement**			
		Present and accurate		
		Location and orientation		
		Superimposition		
3.	**Collimation and shielding**			
4.	**Patient artifacts**			
5.	**Imaging equipment, handling, or processing artifacts**			
6.	**Image sharpness, magnification, minification, and distortion**			
7.	**Positioning**			
	Film size and part/receptor alignment	Appropriate imaging plate size		
		Correct central ray placement		
	Angle	Tube/part angle is correct		
	Rotation	Part rotated correctly		
	Inclusion	All anatomy included		
8.	**Exposure**			
	kVp	Appropriate for type and amount of contrast		
	Scale of contrast	Black/white ratio appropriate		
	Density	Overall too dark/too light		
		Exposure index appropriate		
		mAs selection appropriate		
9.	**Equipment**	Reader error		
		Histogram error		
10.	**Accept/reject**			

Comments/action

_____
_____
_____
_____
_____
_____
_____
_____

FIGURE 12-2 Sample image analysis/reject form.

be used to gently wipe debris off the imaging plate surface. A camel hair brush can be used but should be stored so that dust and dirt do not collect on it. If this is ineffective, cleaning solutions can be used. Use only cleaning solutions specifically recommended by the manufacturer and be sure to follow the Material Safety Data Sheet (MSDS) guidelines provided by the cleaning solution distributor. If the artifact cannot be removed, the imaging plate will have to be replaced.

Imaging plate disposal

Imaging plates contain a small amount of barium, which must be discarded according to state and U.S. Environmental Protection Agency (EPA) regulations.

Disposal must be handled by a licensed disposal company; no other means of disposal, such as putting it in trash cans, is acceptable. This type of disposal requires an EPA identification number, which is assigned by the state. Be sure to be familiar with disposal regulations.

Artifact identification

Monthly QC of images will help to identify recurring artifacts caused by debris on imaging plates, cassettes, laser lenses, and reader mirrors. Major artifacts should be noted at the time of processing and reported; however, smaller, less intrusive artifacts are sometimes missed and ignored, resulting in long-term problems.

Proper problem reporting procedures will provide a mechanism through which recurring quality trends will emerge. If, for example, several reports are received from a particular room that images are excessively noisy or too light, the room may need to be inspected for system interference or AEC recalibration. These procedures will also help service personnel determine what issues exist based on location and frequency.

Service Personnel Responsibilities

Although specific responsibilities will vary from manufacturer to manufacturer and vendor to vendor, generally speaking service personnel have a duty to the consumer to ensure that equipment is being maintained properly. This is accomplished through a program of preventative maintenance that typically takes place semiannually. **Preventative maintenance (PM)** consists of a series of equipment tests that are performed by a service engineer. This engineer may be employed by the hospital or the equipment manufacturer.

Physicist Responsibilities for PSP Systems

Schedules for physicist review of photostimulable phosphor (PSP) digital imaging systems may vary depending on availability (see Box 12-4). One physicist may handle multiple medical facilities, visiting each one on a weekly or monthly basis. Others may be employed by only one facility and be much more active in determining review procedures. Typical responsibilities include the following:

> **BOX 12-4** | **Summary of Physicist Responsibilities**
>
> Semiannual/annual QC for PSP systems
> Component inventory
> Imaging plate dark noise and uniformity
> Exposure indicator calibration accuracy
> System linearity and autoranging response
> Laser beam function
> Limiting resolution and resolution uniformity
> Noise and low-contrast resolution
> Spatial distance accuracy
> Erasure thoroughness
> Aliasing/grid response
> Imaging plate throughput
> Acceptance criteria and quantitative relationships
> Image processing: look-up table transforms and frequency enhancement

- Semi-annual/annual
- Review of departmental images to:
  - Reestablish baseline values
  - Check exposure indicator accuracy with calibrated ion chamber
  - Determine exposure trends
  - Analyze repeat rates
  - Review QC records
  - Analyze service history

The standard QC tests for filtration, collimation, focal-spot size, kVp calibration, exposure timer accuracy, exposure linearity, exposure reproducibility, and protective apparel will remain the same, but the American Association of Physicists in Medicine has established a set of QC parameters to be followed for PSP systems in AAPM Report #93. This report details the tests and reports to be performed. Consult the AAPM website for the most up-to-date QC procedures for digital projection radiography systems.

SUMMARY

- Maintenance of equipment, image acquisition, and processing standards are quality control issues that fit into the concept of total quality management (TQM) or continuous quality improvement (CQI).
- The radiologic technologist is the first line of defense in preventing, recognizing, and reporting quality control (QC) issues.
- Radiologic technologists, service personnel, and radiation physicists each have a set of QC activities that they are responsible to maintain.

CHAPTER REVIEW QUESTIONS

1. What organization developed the standards for acceptance testing and quality control of photostimulable storage phosphor (PSP) imaging systems?
   a. American College of Radiologists
   b. American Society of Radiologic Technologists
   c. American Association of Physicists in Medicine
   d. The Joint Commission

2. Which of the following are daily QC duties of a technologist?
   a. Hinge and latch inspection
   b. Erasure of imaging plates
   c. Image inspection for artifacts
   d. All of the above

3. An imaging plate should be erased when it has not been used for an extended period of time.
   a. True
   b. False

4. Which of the following are weekly QC duties of a technologist?
   a. Clean imaging plates
   b. Clean air intake on reader
   c. Perform a reject analysis
   d. All of the above

5. The EPA regulates the disposal of PSP imaging plates.
   a. True
   b. False

6. The physicist is responsible for performing the preventative maintenance on the digital imaging systems.
   a. True
   b. False

7. How often does a physicist perform an accuracy test between the exposure indices and the ion chamber?
   a. Monthly
   b. Quarterly
   c. Semiannually
   d. Annually

8. Which of the following should not be used to clean the PSP imaging plates?
   a. Camel hair brush
   b. Photographic lens cloth
   c. Corrosive solution
   d. All of the above

9. The display monitors should be cleaned on a monthly basis.
   a. True
   b. False

10. Whose responsibility is it to maintain the quality of digital images?
    a. Technologist
    b. Radiologist
    c. Physicist
    d. All of the above

acceptance testing testing that occurs to ensure equipment or processes are functioning within acceptable limits.

active-matrix plat-panel imager (AMFPI) a flat-panel array with an x-ray absorption material that can be either a photoconductor or a scintillator.

air kerma kinetic energy released per unit mass; measures (in joules) radiation energy that is absorbed in a unit of air.

aliasing loss of digital information because of a fluctuating signal; also known as foldover, biasing, or wraparound.

amplification noise variations in computer chip response to stimulation causing statistical differences between inoperable, fully operable, or inefficient performance.

application service provider (ASP) company that provides outsourcing of archiving and management functions for a pay-per-use or pay-per-month charge.

archive historical collection of images stored in a picture archiving and communication system (PACS).

archive query software function that allows historical information to be gathered from digital storage, such as multiple examinations, a range of dates, or by pathology.

archive server consists of the physical storage device of the archive system; it commonly consists of two or three tiers of storage.

artifacts avoidable extraneous information on the image that interferes or distracts from image quality.

aspect ratio ratio of the width of the monitor to the height of the monitor.

automatic rescaling occurs when exposure is greater or less than the optimal amount to produce a diagnostic image; it is the effort of the computer to "fix" exposure errors.

backing layer soft polymer that protects the back of the cassette.

barcode label label attached either to the cassette or to the imaging plate that identifies the plate for the purpose of matching the examination to the plate.

barium fluorohalide family of photostimulable storage phosphors that can be used in indirect capture systems; most often found in a cassette-based system.

basic input/output system (BIOS) contains a simple set of instructions for the computer to perform several basic functions, such as boot up, run hardware diagnostics, interpret keyboard signals, and so on.

binary code machine language of 1s and 0s.

bit single unit of data.

bit depth the number of bits stored per pixel; defines the shades of gray available for each pixel.

blooming effect an overflow of electrons in a detector element.

brightness level of intensity of a digital image on a display monitor.

bucket brigade scheme process of electron movement during image processing; voltage gates within detector elements are closed, allowing electrons to flow by rows and down by columns to readout row.

burner device that burns data onto a CD or DVD.

bus series of connections, controllers, and chips that creates the information highway of the computer.

bus topology type of network setup in which each of the computers and network devices is connected to a single cable.

byte made up of 8 bits and is the amount of memory needed to store one alphanumeric character.

cassette rigid plastic housing for the imaging plate.

central processing unit (CPU) small chip found on the motherboard that manipulates data sent from a program; brains of the computer.

cesium iodide (CsI) scintillator newer type of amorphous silicon detector that uses a cesium iodide (CsI) scintillator; the scintillator is made by growing very thin crystalline needles (5 μm wide) that work as light-directing tubes, much like fiber optics.

charge-coupled device (CCD) A photosensitive receptor and electronics embedded into a substrate material in a silicon chip; coupling devices that act as cameras.

client-based network similar to a server-based network, in that there is a centralized computer that controls the operations of the network, but rather than sending the entire original resource to the client for processing, the server processes the resource as requested by the client and returns only the results back to the client.

client/server-based system PACS work flow where the images are sent directly to the archive server after acquisition and are centrally located.

coaxial cable network communication medium that is similar to TV cable wiring; type of wire that consists of a center wire surrounded by insulation and a grounded shield of braided wire; the shield minimizes electrical and radio frequency interference.

collimation reduction of the area of beam that reaches the patient through the use of two pairs of lead shutters encased in a housing attached to the x-ray tube.

color layer located between the active layer and the support that absorbs the stimulating light but reflects emitted light.

complementary metal oxide semiconductor (CMOS) special type of memory chip that uses a small rechargeable or lithium battery to retain information about the personal computer's hardware while the computer is turned off; uses a scintillator that, when struck with x-ray photons, converts the x-rays into light photons and stores them in capacitors. Each pixel or detector element has its own amplifier, which is switched on and off by circuitry within the pixel, converting the light photons into electrical charges.

computed radiography (CR) was traditionally the description for cassette-based digital radiography, which is the digital acquisition modality that uses storage phosphor plates to produce projection images; the industry is moving away from using this term.

computer programmable electronic device that can store, retrieve, and process data.

conductive layer layer of material that will absorb and reduce static electricity.

continuous quality improvement (CQI) alternative set of terms for total quality management that includes maintenance of equipment, image acquisition, and processing standards.

contrast manipulation conversion of the digital image using contrast enhancement parameters.

contrast resolution ability of a digital system to display changes in grayscale values.

critical frequency the frequency of a signal that exactly matches the Nyquist frequency, resulting in a zero-amplitude signal caused by phase shifts.

dark current noise operation of the charge-coupled device (CCD) chip without radiation stimulation; caused by elevated temperature.

detective quantum efficiency (DQE) measurement of how efficiently a system converts an x-ray input signal into a useful output image.

detector size actual physical size, length and width, of the x-ray detector.

deviation index the difference between actual exposure and target exposure expressed as a logarithm.

DICOM digital imaging and communications in medicine; it is a global information technology standard that allows network communication between a modality and a PACS.

digital imaging any imaging acquisition process that produces an electronic image that can be viewed and manipulated on a computer.

digital radiography (DR) was traditionally the description for cassette-less systems that use an x-ray absorber material coupled to a flat-panel detector or a charge-coupled device to form the image; the industry is moving away from using this term because it is too broad.

digital versatile disk (DVD) digital storage device that can hold up to seven times more than the CD, which equates to about 9.4 (single-sided) to 17 GB (double-sided) of data; in a DVD, there are multiple layers of the polycarbonate plastic.

direct conversion conversion of x-ray energy to electrical signals without the light-conversion step.

disaster recovery complete copy of the archive housed in another location and immediately available if the front-line archive goes down for any reason.

display workstation generally a display monitor where postprocessing occurs or where images can be viewed.

distributed system PACS work flow where the acquisition modalities send the images to a designated reading station and possibly review stations.

dopants impurities added to a semiconductor to increase conductivity.

dose creep an increasing amount of dose per examination over a period of time that occurs when a technologist sets technical factors, particularly mAs, higher than necessary to avoid exposure errors.

dot pitch measurement of how close the dots are located to one another within a pixel.

dry imager printer that uses heat to develop the film.

dynamic range the ability of an imaging system to respond to varying levels of exposure.

edge enhancement enhancement occurs when fewer pixels in the neighborhood are included in the signal average; the smaller the neighborhood, the greater the enhancement.

error maintenance correction to equipment after errors have occurred.

exposure index the amount of exposure received by the image receptor, not the patient.

exposure indicator number numerical representation of the amount of exposure, usually the mean value.

fast scan direction movement of the laser across the imaging place.

fiber optic cable network communication medium that uses glass threads to transmit data on the network in the form of light.

field effect transistor (FET) device within an imaging detector that isolates each pixel element and reacts like a switch to send the electrical charges to the image processor.

file room workstation workstation found in the radiology file room that may be used to burn CDs or print films for outside use.

film digitizer device that scans hardcopy x-ray images and converts them to digital images.

flat-panel detector detector that consists of a photoconductor, which holds a charge on its surface that can then be read out by a thin-film transistor.

focused grid grid in which the scatter absorbing lead lines are tilted so that, at a prescribed distance, the lines will converge.

gain calibration also known as flat-fielding, this is a process for removal of unwanted densities that interfere with diagnostic image information.

grid frequency number of grid lines per inch.

grid ratio ratio of the height of the grid line to the width of the interspace material.

hanging protocol how a set of images will be displayed on the monitor.

hard drive main repository for programs and documents on the computer.

high-pass filtering technique for the enhancement of contrast and edge that amplifies the frequencies of areas of interest that are known (those frequencies that can be amplified) and suppresses frequencies outside the area of interest.

histogram graphic representation of all of the digitally recorded signals of a digital x-ray exposure.

HL-7 Health Level 7; standard protocol used for medical data systems.

hospital information system (HIS) information system used throughout the hospital; includes direct patient care information, billing systems, and reporting systems.

image annotation software function that allows text or markers to be digitally added to an image.

image lag   a buildup of information resulting from leftover signal or exposures in rapid sequence.

image manager   contains the master database of everything that is in the archive.

image orientation   identification of the top or side of an image.

image sampling   amount of information gathered from pixel storage.

image stitching   process of "sewing" together multiple images to form one continuous image.

image storage   process of sending the digital image to a PACS or CD.

imaging plate   thin piece of plastic with several layers of material that capture and store image data.

indicated equivalent air kerma (K$_{IND}$)   measurement of radiation incident on the image receptor derived from pixel values produced by the exposure to an image receptor.

indirect conversion   two-step process in which x-ray photons are converted to light and then the light photons are converted to an electrical signal.

kVp   kilovoltage peak.

laser   light amplification of stimulated emission of radiation, a device that creates and amplifies a narrow, intense beam of coherent light.

latitude   amount of error that can be made in exposure factor choice and still result in the capture of a quality image.

local area network (LAN)   small area networked with a series of cables or wireless access points so that the computers can share information and devices on the same network.

look-up table (LUT)   reference histogram of the luminance values derived during image acquisition.

low-pass filtering   result of averaging each pixel's frequency with surrounding pixel values to remove high-frequency noise; the result is a reduction of noise and contrast; useful for viewing small structures such as fine bone.

magnetic disk storage   short-term magnetic disk storage, usually found in redundant arrays of independent disks (RAID).

magneto-optical disk (MOD)   very similar to a CD or DVD in that it is read optically with a laser, but the disk itself is housed within a plastic cartridge.

magnification   enlargement of an image in all dimensions without loss of sharpness.

manual send   computer function that allows images to be sent to specified reading stations.

mAs   milliampere-seconds.

matrix   rectangular or square table of numbers that represent the pixel intensity to be displayed on the monitor.

memory   used to store information being currently processed within the central processing unit.

mesh topology   network that has multiple pathway interconnecting devices and networks.

modulation transfer function   ability of a system to record available spatial frequencies.

moiré   grid line or image noise pattern that occurs either when the alignment of the grid to the laser scan direction is incorrect or when spatial frequency is greater than the Nyquist frequency; a wraparound image will result.

motherboard   largest circuitry board inside the computer; it contains many important small components to make the computer function properly.

multiple manual selection mode   area of interest is selected by the technologist, and the image is derived from the selected areas imaged in semiautomatic mode.

navigation functions   options available on the workstation that allow movement through menus, menu options, and image processing choices, as well as movement through a series or stack of images and/or patient image folders.

network   two or more objects sharing resources and information; interconnected computers, terminals, and servers connected by communication channels sharing data and program resources.

network bridge   created so that larger networks can be segmented or broken up into smaller networks to reduce traffic within that network.

network hub central meeting point where cables from several devices can come together and share information throughout the group; it is a simple boxlike device with several wiring ports available to receive and pass on data to various pieces of equipment; the hub sends all information to every device connected.

network interface card (NIC) interface between the computer and the network medium.

network protocol agreed-on set of rules for network communication.

network router device that can read portions of the messages and direct them to their intended target, even if the device is on a separate network and uses a different network protocol.

network switch similar to a hub, but it sends data only to those devices to which the data are directed.

noise any type of signal interference in a digital image.

noise power spectrum spatial frequency content and spatial characteristics of noise.

Nyquist theorem when sampling a signal such as the conversion from an analog to a digital image, the sampling frequency must be greater than twice the bandwidth of the input signal so that the reconstruction of the original image will be nearly perfect.

operating system software that controls the computer hardware and acts as a bridge between applications and the hardware.

PACS picture archiving and communication system; consists of digital acquisition, display workstations, and storage devices interconnected through a network.

PACS administrator the person trained to oversee the PACS.

patient demographics input information regarding patient age, identifying number, ordering physician, and so on.

peer-to-peer network each computer on the network is considered equal; no computer has ultimate control over another.

phosphor center area within the phosphor layer where electrons are trapped.

phosphor layer layer of photostimulable phosphor that "traps" electrons during exposure; usually made of phosphors from the barium fluorohalide family (e.g., barium fluorohalide, chlorohalide, or bromohalide crystals).

photoconductor a material that absorbs x-rays and in turn emits an electrical charge.

photometer device used to measure the luminescence of areas on the monitor.

photomultiplier electronic device that amplifies light energy.

photostimulable luminescence (PSL) light produced by a phosphor when struck by light or x-ray photons.

photostimulable phosphor (PSP) phosphor that produces light when stimulated by light or x-ray photons.

picture archiving and communication system (PACS) networked group of computers, servers, and archives that can be used to manage digital images.

pixel basic picture element on a display.

port collection of connectors sticking out of the back of the computer that link adapter cards, drives, printers, scanners, keyboards and mice, and other peripherals that may be used.

power supply delivers all electricity and provides connections to power devices in the computer.

preventative maintenance (PM) periodic testing of equipment and materials before problem occurrence.

protective layer very thin, tough, clear plastic covering in the imaging plate for protection of the phosphor layer.

quality assurance (QA) another term, now considered antiquated, for quality management; typically focuses on the person rather than the process.

quality control (QC) subdivision of quality management that focuses on equipment functions.

quality control (QC) workstation dedicated computer and monitor for the purpose of reviewing digital images.

quantum mottle failure of an imaging system to record densities; usually caused by a lack of x-ray photons.

quantum efficiency the absolute efficiency of the light signal and created signal in a digital imaging system.

quantum noise recording error in the digital image.

radiology information system (RIS) information system used in the radiology department for ordering examinations and reporting results.

raster zigzag electron scanning pattern.

reading workstation computer and monitor generally used by the physician interpreting the digital images.

redundant array of independent disks (RAID) composed of several magnetic disks or hard drives that are linked together in an array.

reflective layer layer in the imaging plate that sends light in a forward direction when released in the cassette reader; this may be black to reduce the spread of stimulating light and the escape of emitted light; some detail is lost in this process.

refresh rate measure of how fast the monitor rewrites the screen or the number of times that the image is redrawn on the display each second.

resolution number of pixels contained on a display.

review workstation workstation used by other health care personnel to view radiology images.

ring topology network in which the devices are connected in a circle.

routine maintenance synonymous with preventive maintenance; maintenance of equipment that occurs before problem occurrences.

scintillators structured or unstructured phosphor arrays that emit light when stimulated by x-rays.

server computer that manages resources for other computers, servers, and networked devices.

server-based network network in which a centralized computer (server) controls the operations, files, and sometimes the programs of the computers (clients) attached to the network.

shuttering used to blacken out the white collimation borders in a digital image, effectively eliminating veil glare.

signal-to-noise ratio the ratio of the amount of total signal versus the amount of noise present in any digital image.

slow scan direction movement of the imaging plate through the reader; also known as translation or subscan direction.

smoothing also known as low-pass filtering, the result of averaging each pixel's frequency with surrounding pixel values to remove high-frequency noise.

softcopy reading images on the computer without hardcopy films.

sound card a computer board that contains the circuitry for recording and reproducing sound on a personal computer.

spatial frequency resolution amount of detail or sharpness in a digital image.

spectrum sensitivity the range of light sensitivity (wavelength) of a charge-coupled device.

speed in conventional radiography, *speed* is determined by the size and layers of crystals in the film and screen; computed radiography system "speeds" are a reflection of the amount of photostimulable luminescence given off by the imaging plate while being scanned by the laser.

standardized radiation exposure (K_{STD}) standard exposure typical of an imaging receptor system that is made with additional filtration to simulate patient tissue.

star topology network that has the devices connected to a central hub or switch.

statistical noise noise resulting from a lack of light photon emission from the scintillator.

structured phosphor needlelike, highly organized phosphor crystals.

super user someone trained within the hospital to help troubleshoot and teach others to use the PACS.

support layer semirigid material in the imaging plate that gives the imaging sheet some strength.

system architecture hardware and software infrastructure of the system's work flow.

tape magnetic tape cartridges used for long-term storage archives.

target equivalent air kerma value (K_TGT) a set of established values that represent optimal exposures for each specific body part and view.

teleradiology moving images via telephone lines to and from remote locations.

The Joint Commission (TJC) organization that accredits health care organizations, such as hospitals, clinics, and labs.

thick client computer that can work independently from the network and can process and manage its own files.

thin-film transistor (TFT) photosensitive array, made up of small (about 100 to 200 μm) pixels; converts the light into electrical charges.

thin client device that is found on a network that requests services and resources from a server.

tier level, layer, or division of something.

tomosynthesis digital image slice acquisition in sequence; similar to tomography but allows for image reconstruction.

topology physical (geometric) layout of the connected devices on a network.

total quality management (TQM) see *continuous quality improvement*.

twisted-pair wire network communication medium that consists of four twisted pairs of copper wire that are insulated and bundled together with an RJ-45 termination.

ultra density optical disk (UDO) new generation MOD; uses blue laser technology in its read and write activities.

unstructured phosphor small randomly shaped and bound crystals, also known as a turbid phosphor (powered granules).

viewable area measured from one corner of the display to the opposite corner diagonally.

web-based system very similar to a client/server system with regard to how the data flow, but the biggest difference is that not only are the images held centrally, but so is the application software for the client display.

wet imager printer that uses chemicals to develop the film.

wide area network (WAN) network that spans a large area, city, state, nation, continent, and/or world.

window level image manipulation parameter that changes screen image brightness, usually through the use of a mouse.

window width image manipulation parameter that changes screen image contrast, usually through the use of a mouse.

wireless network communication medium that uses either infrared or radio frequencies as its means of communication.

work flow amount of work or examinations completed over a period of time.

µGy	microgray	DQE	detector quantum efficiency
µm	micrometer	DR	digital radiography
2D	two-dimensional	DSA	digital subtraction angiography
3D	three-dimensional	DVD	digital versatile disk
AAPM	American Association of Physicists in Medicine	EI	exposure index
		EMR	electronic medical record
AC	alternating current	EPA	Environmental Protection Agency
ACR	American College of Radiology		
ADC	analog-to-digital converter	eV	electron volt
AEC	automatic exposure control	FET	field effect transistor
AGP	accelerated graphics port	FOV	field of view
AIT	advanced intelligent tape	FPD	flat-panel detector
AMFPI	active-matrix flat-panel imager	Gd$_2$O$_2$S	gadolinium oxysulphide
ANSI	American National Standards Institute	GB	gigabyte
		GUI	graphical user interface
AP	anteroposterior	HIPAA	Health Insurance Portability and Accountability Act
a-Se	amorphous selenium		
a-Si:H	hydrogenated amorphous silicon	HIS	hospital information system
ASP	application service provider	HL-7	Health Level 7
BIOS	basic input/output system	Hz	hertz
C7-T1	refers to the junction of the seventh cervical vertebra and the first thoracic vertebra	ID	identification
		IDE	integrated drive electronics
		IP	Internet protocol
CAD	computer-aided diagnosis	IP	image plate
cat 5	category 5	JPEG	joint photographic expert group
CCD	charge-coupled device	keV	kilo-electron-volt
CD	compact disk	kVp	kilovoltage peak (prime)
cm	centimeter	L	latitude
CMOS	complementary metal oxide semiconductor	L5/S1	refers to the junction of the fifth lumbar vertebra and the first section of the sacrum
CPU	central processing unit		
CQI	continuous quality management	LAN	local area network
CR	computed radiography	LCD	liquid crystal display
CRT	cathode ray tube	lgM	logarithm
CsI	cesium iodide	lp/mm	line pairs per millimeter
CsI(TI)	thallium doped cesium iodide	LTO	linear tape open
CT	computed tomography	LUT	look-up table
DAS	direct attached storage	mAs	milliampere-seconds
DC	direct current	MB	megabyte
del	detector element	MAN	metropolitan area network
DICOM	digital imaging and communications in medicine	MIDI	musical instrument digital interface
DLT	digital linear tape	MIP	maximum intensity projection

MOD	magneto-optical disk	RAID	redundant array of independent disks
mp	megapixel	RAM	random access memory
MPR	multiplanar reconstruction	RF	radio frequency
MP3	moving picture experts group audio layer 3	RIS	radiology information system
mR	milliroentgen	ROM	read-only memory
MRI	magnetic resonance imaging	RW	read and write many times
MS-DOS	Microsoft–Disk Operating System	S (number)	sensitivity
MSDS	material data safety sheets	SAN	storage area network
MTF	modulation transfer function	SCP	service class provider
NAS	network attached storage	SCSI	small computer system interface
NEMA	National Electrical Manufacturers Association	SCU	service class user
NIC	network interface card	SDO	Standards Developing Organization
nm	nanometer	SMPTE	Society of Motion Pictures and Television Engineers
NPS	noise power spectrum	SOPs	service/object pairs
OID	object image distance	SQL	structured query language
OLED	organic light emitting diode	SSD	shaded surface display
OS	operating system	TB	terabyte
PA	posteroanterior	TCP	transmission control protocol
PACS	picture archiving and communication system	TFT	thin-film transistor
PC	personal computer	TJC	The Joint Commission
PCI	peripheral component interconnect	TQM	total quality management
PM	preventative maintenance	UDO	ultra density optical disk
PSL	photostimulable luminescence	UID	unique identifiers
PSP	photostimulable storage phosphor	USB	universal serial bus
PS2	IBM programming system 2	VA	Veterans Administration
QA	quality assurance	VRT	volume rendering technique
QC	quality control	W	watt
		WAN	wide area network
		WAV	waveform audio
		WORM	write once–read many

Page numbers followed by "f" indicate figures, "t" indicate tables, and "b" indicate boxes.